CASE STUDIES IN

IMMUNOLOGY

CASE STUDIES IN

IMMUNOLOGY

Ivan M Roitt MA DSc(Oxon) Hon MRCP(Lond) FRCPath FRS
Emeritus Professor of Immunology
Director of the Institute of Biomedical Science
University College London Medical School
London, UK

Jonathan Brostoff MA DM(Oxon) DSc FRCP FRCPath
Reader in Clinical Immunology
Department of Immunology
University College London Medical School
London, UK

David K Male MA PhD
Senior Lecturer in Neuroimmunology
Department of Neuropathology
Institute of Psychiatry
London, UK

Alexander Gray BSc(Hons)
Department of Immunology
University College London Medical School
London, UK

M Mosby

Copyright © 1994 Times Mirror International Publishers Limited
Published in 1994 by Mosby–Wolfe, an imprint of Times Mirror International Publishers Limited
Printed by Grafos S.A. Arte sobre papel, Barcelona, Spain
ISBN 0 7234 2052 1

For full details of all Times Mirror International Publishers Limited titles please write to Times Mirror International Publishers Limited, Lynton House, 7–12 Tavistock Square, London WC1H 9LB, England.

A CIP catalogue record for this book is available from the British Library.

Preface

This book of case studies is designed to put basic immunological mechanisms into a clinical perspective. In a textbook of basic science it may seem inappropriate, and indeed difficult to use clinical case studies as illustrative material. However, immunology is relevant and indeed central to many disease processes in both animals and man, thus supporting this approach.

Even if you, the reader, are not planning a career in medicine, we hope that these case studies will provide you with a further perspective on the wide variety of immune-related diseases whose basic immunological mechanisms are described in *Immunology,* 3rd edn.

Jonathan Brostoff
Alexander Gray

Contents

The page and chapter numbers cited at
the top of each answer page refer to
Roitt *et al. Immunology,* 3rd edn
(Mosby, 1993)

chapter 1

Immunity to Viruses, Bacteria, and Fungi

CASE 1

At 13 years of age, Stephen, who was a bicycle freak, was involved in an accident. He was knocked off his bike and suffered a number of cuts and bruises, including bruising over his left loin. He was taken to hospital because of probable concussion and was monitored closely. That night he complained of abdominal pain and it was noticed that his blood pressure had dropped precipitously. Transfusion was arranged, but even five units of blood was not enough to maintain his blood pressure. He was taken to the operating theatre and laparotomy revealed a ruptured spleen, which was removed. His postoperative course was uneventful.

Ten years later at 23 years of age, Stephen developed a cough, which was associated with left lower chest pain. Within a day he had a high temperature and when seen by his doctor had a low blood pressure and was obviously unwell. He was admitted to hospital where blood cultures grew *Streptococcus pneumoniae*. Antibiotics were given immediately. After a stormy course he recovered.

QUESTIONS

1 What are the major functions of the spleen?
2 What is Stephen's clearance of antibody-coated autologous red cells likely to be?
3 Are specific immunisations advisable following splenectomy?
4 Are there likely to be any immunoglobulin or other serum component abnormalities following splenectomy?

NOTES FOR REVISION

YOUR ANSWERS

1 Major functions of the spleen

2 Clearance of antibody-coated autologous red cells

3 Specific immunisations advisable following splenectomy

4 Immunoglobulin or other serum component abnormalities following splenectomy

CASE 1

pp. 3.3–3.4, 15.11–15.13

ANSWERS

1 Major functions of the spleen

Opsonisation and production of IgG2 antibody. Bacteria with a capsule are cleared by the spleen. The dose of organisms that can cause an infection is much smaller in people after a splenectomy because such people have a reduced amount of phagocytic tissue.

2 Clearance of antibody-coated autologous red cells

Antibody-coated red blood cells are cleared much more quickly than uncoated cells. The Fc is bound to phagocytic cells in the spleen. Such binding is more avid if C3 is also fixed. Removing a major phagocytic organ must therefore alter handling of opsonised organisms and reduce this clearance.

3 Specific immunisations advisable following splenectomy

Despite an increased risk of infection with encapsulated bacteria following splenectomy, there are no national guidelines in the UK regarding immun-isation or antibiotic prophylaxis. Some 50% of all infections in these patients are caused by *Streptococcus pneumoniae* and the administration of a vaccine consisting of capsular polysaccharides derived from pathogenic pneumococcal strains has been advocated for some time. Recent recommendations also include *Haemophilus influenzae* type b (Hib) and meningococcal A and C vaccines.

4 Immunoglobulin or other serum component abnormalities following splenectomy

IgG2 and IgM may be low as well as various complement components.

CASE 2

Mr Quinn, a 59-year-old man, underwent elective sigmoid colectomy for recurrent diverticular disease. He had no other medical history of note and was fit and well before the operation. The procedure was carried out without incident and his immediate postoperative recovery was uneventful. Two days after surgery he became confused and was difficult to rouse.

On examination he had a temperature of 38.5°C and a thready radial pulse of 125 beats/min. His blood pressure had dropped to 100/70 mm Hg and his jugular venous pulse was not visible. His peripheral pulses were all present, but his extremities felt cold. Examination of his abdomen was unremarkable and the wound was healing well with no signs of infection.

On investigation his white cell count was $18 \times 10^9/l$, haemoglobin 11.8 g/dl, and platelet count $130 \times 10^9/l$. Serum creatinine was mildly elevated. Samples of blood and urine were taken for culture, and he was started on cefuroxime, metronidazole, and gentamicin for suspected septicaemia. Intravenous colloid was given to correct his hypovolaemia.

Over the next 12 hours his condition deteriorated. He became tachypnoeic and drifted into a semiconscious state. On examination he had widespread respiratory crackles and a radial pulse of 135 beats/min. His blood pressure dropped to 90/50 mm Hg. Arterial blood gas measurements showed a PaO_2 of 7.8 kPa and a $PaCO_2$ of 6.2 kPa on 60% oxygen by mask. He was immediately admitted to the intensive care unit.

On arrival in intensive care he was intubated and intermittent positive pressure ventilation was commenced. Further colloid was administered for hypovolaemia and a pulmonary artery inflation catheter was inserted into the pulmonary artery. A chest radiograph showed bilateral lung infiltrates.

A diagnosis of adult respiratory distress syndrome (ARDS) was made based on a history of sepsis, a low PaO_2, a non-raised pulmonary artery wedge pressure, and the bilateral radiological lung infiltrates.

Intravenous colloids failed to improve Mr Quinn's blood pressure, and he was started on dobutamine and noradrenaline. Intravenous dopamine was given to improve renal and splanchnic perfusion and a cause for his septicaemia was sought. A plain abdominal radiograph and an ultrasound scan did not reveal any abnormality. At laparotomy purulent fluid was found in the peritoneal cavity and the colorectal anastomosis had broken down. A defunctioning colostomy and peritoneal lavage was performed and Mr Quinn was readmitted to intensive care. Three days postoperatively he developed a secondary chest infection and died shortly afterwards. Blood, urine, and wound swab cultures were all negative, but a culture of peritoneal fluid grew *Escherichia coli* and *Streptococcus faecalis*, both of which are normal bowel commensal bacteria.

QUESTIONS

1 What are endotoxins?
2 How do endotoxins mediate their effects?
3 What conditions are associated with ARDS?
4 What is the immunopathology of ARDS?

NOTES FOR REVISION

YOUR ANSWERS

1 **What are endotoxins?**

2 **How endotoxins mediate their effects**

3 **Conditions associated with ARDS**

4 **Immunopathology of ARDS**

CASE 2

pp.15.8–15.9

ANSWERS

1 What are endotoxins?

Endotoxins are structural components of Gram-negative cell walls, which are only liberated following cell death or lysis. They are complexes of phospholipids and polysaccharides, usually termed bacterial lipopolysaccharides (LPS). Their antigenicity varies, but their biological effects are the same.

2 How endotoxins mediate their effects

Unlike exotoxins, endotoxins exhibit only weak antigenicity, but are still able to injure the parenchyma of various organs in severe sepsis. More significantly they are responsible for the activation of primed macrophages, which are important mediators of septic shock. Macrophages release tumour necrosis factor (TNF), which acts on polymorphs and macrophages to mediate aggregation and adhesion to endothelial cells. Furthermore TNF stimulates the release of platelet activating factor (PAF), which causes platelet aggregation, and is responsible for increasing IL-1 production from macrophages and endothelial cells, increasing capillary 'leakiness' to inflammatory cells.

Endotoxins also have a direct effect on neutrophils by increasing lysosomal production and discharge, and activate Factor XII therefore triggering the coagulation pathway. Both the classical and alternative complement cascades are also initiated. This results in vasodilatation, hypotension, and poor organ perfusion. Diffuse intravascular coagulation can also occur.

3 Conditions associated with ARDS

The following often precede ARDS:
- Sepsis (bacteraemia, septicaemia)
- Trauma (head injuries, fat emboli)
- Localised infection (pneumonia)
- Aspiration (gastric contents, sea or fresh water)
- Haematological (diffuse intravascular coagulation, repeated blood transfusion)
- Metabolic disorders (pancreatitis, uraemia)
- Others (inhaled toxins, drug overdose, radiation)

4 Immunopathology of ARDS

It is believed that ARDS is triggered by an initial 'insult' related to one or more of the conditions listed above. Endotoxin liberation and/or complement activation result in macrophage activation and the release of TNF and IL-1. These have a variety of effects on different cellular and enzyme systems.
- **Effect on neutrophils**: release of protease inhibitors, increased adherence and aggregation, and liberation of free oxygen radical scavengers.
- **Effect on platelets**: release of prostacyclin and platelet aggregation and activation.
- **Effect on endothelium**: increased permeability and production of nitric oxide, increased arachidonic acid metabolism and release of prostaglandins, thromboxanes, and leukotrienes.
- **Activation of the coagulation pathway** with inhibition of fibrinolysis leading to the formation of microthrombi.

These factors combine to produce interstitial and alveolar oedema with extravasation of red blood cells. The endothelium and epithelium become damaged with sloughing of the cells lining the alveoli. Surfactant production is decreased following damage to the Type II pneumocyte by the release of proteolytic enzymes. The result is alveolar filling or closure leading to a reduced functional residual capacity and reduced compliance.

CASE 3

John, a six-year-old schoolboy, presented in the Accident & Emergency Dept. (A&E) with a two-day history of malaise, fever, blood in his urine, and a puffy face. He had no history of renal disease or abdominal trauma. Past medical history of note was a sore throat some twelve days before, which had settled without a visit to his general practitioner. His mother remembered that he had received the standard immunisation schedule.

On examination John was febrile, had periorbital and ankle oedema, and his blood pressure was 130/90 mm Hg. The skin on his face and trunk was peeling and he had a reddened tongue. The rest of the examination was unremarkable. Results of investigations are shown in Fig. 1.1.

Fig. 1.1 Results of investigations

Investigation	Result
Urine analysis	Macroscopic haematuria, moderate proteinuria and granular casts
Glomerular filtration rate (measured by creatinine clearance)	Reduced
Urine culture	Negative
Culture from a throat swab	Positive for *Streptococcus pyogenes*
Serum sample	Positive for antibodies to streptolysin O (ASO), DNAse B and hyaluronidase
Serum C3	Low
C4	Normal
Haemoglobin	Low
White cell count	Normal

A diagnosis of post-streptococcal glomerulonephritis was made and John was started on benzylpenicillin. His fluid retention was controlled by restriction of salt and water intake and loop diuretics. Within a week his blood pressure had dropped to 105/70 mm Hg with no haematuria or proteinuria. Several weeks after presentation his C3 level had returned to normal. At follow-up he was well and had no signs of renal impairment.

QUESTIONS
1 Explain the pathogenesis of acute glomerulonephritis?
2 What is seen if a renal biopsy from this patient is stained with fluorescein conjugated anti-IgG and anti-C3?
3 What is the long-term prognosis of this condition?
4 Are all strains of Group A streptococci equally pathogenic?

NOTES FOR REVISION

YOUR ANSWERS

1 **Pathogenesis of acute glomerulonephritis**

2 **What is seen when the renal biopsy is stained with fluorescein conjugated anti-IgG and anti-C3**

3 **Long-term prognosis**

4 **Pathogenicity of different strains of Group A streptococci**

CASE 3

pp. 15.8, 21.8–21.12

ANSWERS

1 Pathogenesis of acute glomerulonephritis

Post-streptococcal glomerulonephritis can occur at any age, but is most common in male children. The renal symptoms appear some 1–3 weeks after an acute infection with a group A haemolytic streptococcus. Typically the clinical picture is of pharyngitis. Renal biopsy demonstrates acute diffuse proliferative glomerulonephritis. There is diffuse enlargement and increased cellularity of the glomeruli. The cellular changes are a mixture of increased numbers of endothelial and mesangial cells combined with infiltration of neutrophils and macrophages. On electron microscopy there are subepithelial electron-dense granular deposits.

2 What is seen when the renal biopsy is stained with fluorescein conjugated anti-IgG and anti-C3

Immunofluorescence demonstrates that the electron-dense areas consist of deposits of IgG and C3, which strongly suggests that immune complexes are deposited subepithelially. By implication it has been suggested that these complexes are derived from streptococcal antigens and their specific antibodies. Experiments to identify bacterial antigens deposited in the glomeruli have produced conflicting results and it is not clear whether the complexes are formed in the circulation or *in situ*. Low circulating C3 and high anti-ASO antibody titres support an immune complex aetiology.

3 Long-term prognosis

The prognosis is excellent if treatment is given rapidly. The glomeruli usually return to normal within weeks, although the increased number of mesangial cells may persist for some months. It is worth noting that other infectious agents can cause glomerulonephritis: for example, *Staphylococcus aureus*, Epstein–Barr virus, and the malarial parasite.

4 Pathogenicity of different strains of Group A streptococci

Not all strains of Group A streptococci are equally pathogenic. Griffiths types 1, 4, 12, 25, and 49 have been noted to be nephritogenic with the other types not being associated with renal disease. No explanation has yet been found for this.

chapter 2

Tumour Immunology

 CASE 4

Mrs Jones, a 54-year-old lady, was seen in A&E after falling and injuring her right hip. On questioning she noted a six-month history of backache, lethargy, and weakness. She was postmenopausal, but was taking hormone replacement therapy. Past medical history comprised three episodes of pneumococcal pneumonia in the past two years.

On examination Mrs Jones had a swollen, tender, and bruised right hip and one inch of true shortening of the right leg. She was clinically anaemic with pallor of her mucous membranes and nailbeds, and had a mild tachycardia. The rest of her examination was unremarkable. Results of the investigations are shown in Fig. 2.1.

Fig. 2.1 Results of investigations

Investigation	Result
X-ray of pelvis and upper femurs	Fracture of the neck of the femur through an area of decreased bone density
Red cell count	Normocytic, normochromic anaemia
White cell count	Normal
Platelet count	Just below normal range
Erythrocyte sedimentation rate	Raised
Urea and creatinine	Above normal ranges
Serum albumin	Depleted
Liver function tests	Normal
Bone isoenzyme of alkaline phosphatase	Mildly elevated
Serum calcium	Raised

The fracture was managed conservatively and further investigations were performed, as malignancy was suspected (see Fig. 2.2).

Fig. 2.2 Results of further investigations

X-ray of spine and skull	Multiple punched-out lytic lesions
Electrophoresis of serum proteins	A monoclonal peak in the gamma region identified as IgG of the kappa type
Serum IgG	Grossly elevated
IgM and IgA	Low
Immunoelectrophoresis of a monoclonal protein band found in the urine	Kappa Bence–Jones protein
Bone marrow biopsy	Increased numbers of abnormal plasma cells, containing IgG and kappa chains only. A decreased number of remaining plasma cells contained IgM and IgA compared with normal bone marrow cell ratios

A diagnosis of multiple myeloma was made and Mrs Jones was started on a course of chemotherapy.

QUESTIONS

1 What is Bence–Jones protein?
2 What is the pathology of this condition?
3 Why has Mrs Jones had recurrent pneumonia?
4 Why is Mrs Jones anaemic?

YOUR ANSWERS

1 Bence–Jones protein

2 Pathology of multiple myeloma

3 Cause of recurrent pneumonia

4 Cause of anaemia

CASE 4

pp. 4.1–4.7, Chapter 17

ANSWERS

1 Bence–Jones protein

Plasma cells synthesise a larger amount of immunoglobulin light chains than heavy chains. Whole immunoglobulins are not excreted by the kidney because their molecular weight is too high, but light chains are found in the urine. Under normal circumstances, they are polyclonal in specificity, reflecting their synthesis by many specific plasma cells. Bence–Jones proteins are free monoclonal light chains and therefore reflect their origin from a single antigen-specific plasma cell clone. Urinalysis for Bence–Jones protein is performed by concentrating the urine, electrophoresis, and immunofixation.

2 Pathology of multiple myeloma

Multiple myeloma is a neoplastic proliferation of plasma cells or their precursors. Diagnosis is based on three findings:
- Bence-Jones protein in the urine.
- Osteolytic lesions of the bones.
- The presence of increased numbers of abnormal plasma cells or their precursors in the bone marrow.

The malignant proliferation of the cells is responsible for the bone lesions and the excess production of immunoglobulin, which may be IgG (50% of cases), IgA (25%), or light chains only (Bence–Jones myeloma, 20%). IgD and IgE are only rarely involved.

The aetiology and pathogenesis are unknown, but excess IL-6 production has been implicated.

3 Cause of recurrent pneumonia

Patients with multiple myeloma have an increased susceptibility to bacterial infections, particularly pneumococcal pneumonia in the early stages of the disease, and sepsis and Gram-negative urinary tract infections in the later stages. This state is caused by a decrease in the production of normal immunoglobulins of all classes and is believed to originate from suppression of normal plasma cells by the malignancy.

4 Cause of anaemia

Anaemia is found in the majority of patients with multiple myeloma at some point in the course of the disease. It is frequently normocytic and normochromic and is typically refractory to iron, folate, and vitamin B_{12} treatment. The cause of the anaemia is loss of bone marrow to tumour and the suppression of normal marrow by tumour cell secretions. The excess production of light chains is also associated with red cell haemolysis.

chapter 3

Immunodeficiency

■ CASE 5

At three years of age, John developed a painful ear; he was seen by a doctor who diagnosed otitis media and gave him antibiotics. However, in spite of the treatment, his ear drum ruptured and pus was seen in the external auditory meatus. The pain cleared and with the antibiotics the secretions dried up. The drum healed with little scarring. John then had recurrent sore throats, some of which gave a positive culture for bacteria; the relevant antibiotics were given. At seven years of age John had bacterial tonsillitis twice and one episode of bronchitis.

Summer hay fever and pollen asthma were first noticed when he was 10 years old; he had never had atopic eczema. As a result of further episodes of tonsillitis John had a tonsillectomy when he was 11. Subsequently, he suffered several episodes of gastroenteritis, which responded to antibiotic treatment. At this stage the paediatrician could find no clinical abnormality when John was examined, but did find that he had an abnormally low level of IgA.

QUESTIONS

1 What other immunoglobulin abnormalities might be present in John's serum?
2 What other clinical associations are there with IgA deficiency?
3 Is IgA deficiency often asymptomatic, and if so why?
4 Is John likely to have a problem with blood transfusions?

NOTES FOR REVISION

YOUR ANSWERS

1 Other immunoglobulin abnormalities in John's serum

2 Other clinical associations of IgA deficiency

3 Is IgA deficiency often asymptomatic, and if so why?

4 Is John likely to have a problem with blood transfusions?

CASE 5

pp. 1.12, 18.2

ANSWERS

1 Other immunoglobulin abnormalities in John's serum

In the majority of patients, IgA is absent in both serum and secretions, with normal amounts of secretory component and normal T cell function. A small proportion of patients will have normal levels of secretory IgA, but little or none in the serum. There is a group of patients who are also deficient in IgG2 and it is possible that they are more prone to infection.

2 Other clinical associations of IgA deficiency

The increased risk of infection is the main clinical association but allergic disorders affect about 33% of patients, and autoimmune diseases affect a similar proportion. There is certainly a strong association with auto-antibodies, both organ specific and non-organ specific.

3 Is IgA deficiency often asymptomatic, and if so why?

The incidence of IgA deficiency in the general population is difficult to ascertain. It is probable that the majority are asymptomatic. To become symptomatic it may be necessary to have two defects, but the second one has not yet been clearly identified apart from IgG2 deficiency.

4 Is John likely to have a problem with blood transfusions?

For a patient who is absolutely deficient in IgA there is obviously the possibility of developing anti-IgA antibodies. These are unlikely to be present in a child, but patients who have been transfused may well develop such antibodies. In this situation, a transfusion may produce a reaction and it is wise to measure anti-IgA antibodies before any such intervention.

CASE 6

Alex was born at term after an uneventful pregnancy. Delivery was normal and at birth he weighed 4 kg. He did not require any resuscitation and had no anatomical abnormalities. His first few months of life were without incident, but at eight months he developed an upper respiratory tract infection which became complicated by *Haemophilus influenzae* sinusitis. He was treated with chloramphenicol and ampicillin and recovered well. Within a month he was seen again by his doctor with symptoms of otitis media. The causal organism was again identified as *H. influenzae* and he was treated accordingly.

At 12 months Alex was found to have a red, tender, and swollen arm. A diagnosis of cellulitis was made and he was successfully treated with flucloxacillin. At 15 months he was admitted to hospital with severe diarrhoea caused by *Giardia lamblia,* which responded to antibiotic treatment. At this visit his height and weight were noted to be below the third centile. His older sisters aged three and five years had normal growth patterns and no history of recurrent infections.

Alex's mother confirmed that he had received the standard immunisation schedule of diphtheria and tetanus (both toxoids), pertussis (killed *Bordetella pertussis* bacteria), polio (live attenuated polio virus), and measles, mumps, and rubella (all live attenuated organisms). No abnormal reactions had occurred after any immunisation. The results of investigations are shown in Fig. 3.1.

Fig. 3.1 Results of investigations

Investigation	Result
Haemoglobin	Normal
White cell count	Normal
Differential white cell analysis	
Neutrophil, basophil, eosinophil, and monocyte counts	All normal
Total lymphocyte count	Normal
T cell count	Normal
Immature and mature B cell numbers	Very low: almost undetectable
Analysis of immunoglobulin classes	
Serum IgG	Very low 0.3 g/l; (normal 5.5–10.0 g/l)
Serum IgM	Very low 0.02 g/l; (normal 0.4–1.8 g/l)
Serum IgA, IgD, and IgE	Absent
Antibodies made in response to immunisations	Not detected

A diagnosis of X-linked agammaglobulinaemia was made and Alex was started on intravenous IgG replacement therapy. The immunoglobulin was obtained from a large pool of donor serum using ethanol fractionation and administered at 3–4 week intervals. Members of his family were advised to attend for genetic counselling, which was aided by the use of a gene probe test for the deficiency. At a follow-up appointment several years later Alex was well and reported only one chest infection since diagnosis.

QUESTIONS

1 Why was Alex well for the first few months of life?
2 What are the major clinical complications to be expected?
3 How would Alex react to a skin test with BCG?
4 What treatment should be given?

YOUR ANSWERS

1 **Why was Alex well for the first few months of life?**

2 **Major clinical complications**

3 **Reaction to a skin test with BCG**

4 **What treatment should be given?**

CASE 6

pp.11.15, 18.1–18.2

ANSWERS

1 Why was Alex well for the first few months of life?

Trans-placental maternal antibody will provide a level of immunoglobulin that can protect the fetus for some months. Complications are therefore only expected after maternal antibody has disappeared, at which stage the child has little or no humoral protection.

2 Major clinical complications

There are three major complications:
- Arthritis affecting the ankle and knee is common before treatment starts.
- Severe diarrhoea with weight loss in 20% of patients.
- Encephalitis, a severe complication often caused by echovirus 11 and often resistant to treatment with conventional amounts of immunoglobulin.

However, patients handle most forms of viral infection normally and recover well from exanthemata.

3 Reaction to a skin test with BCG

Skin tests for delayed type hypersensitivity should be normal as there is no abnormality in the T-lymphocytes or their function, allowing normal cell-mediated immunity.

4 What treatment should be given?

The most important aspect of treatment is to give replacement with human immune serum globulin. This can be given intramuscularly every two or four weeks depending on the dose. The gammaglobulin can also be given intravenously. A combination of antibiotics, such as trimethoprim and sulphamethoxazole, is useful where there is infection of the upper respiratory tract.

CASE 7

David was born at term after an uneventful pregnancy. At birth he was cyanosed and required oxygen from the first few minutes of life. He was born with abnormal external features including micrognathia, large slanted eyes, and low set prominent ears with notched pinnae. Within the first 36 hours of life he had episodes of muscle tetany.

The results of investigations are shown in Fig. 3.2.

Fig. 3.2 Results of investigations	
Investigation	**Result**
Serum calcium	Below normal range
Serum phosphorus	Elevated
Parathyroid hormone assay	Negative (suggesting parathyroid deficiency as a cause for the low calcium level)
Haemoglobin	Normal
White cell count	Low
Serum levels of IgG, IgM, and IgA	Normal
Chest radiograph	Right-sided aortic arch and an absent thymic shadow
Chromosomal analysis	Deletion on long arm of chromosome 22

Chromosomal analysis by *in situ* hybridisation of gene probes demonstrated a sub-microscopic deletion of the proximal long arm of chromosome 22. A diagnosis of DiGeorge syndrome was made and David's management was continued in a special care baby unit. The tetanic episodes were initially treated with intravenous calcium gluconate and were followed up with a low phosphorus diet, calcium supplements, and high doses of vitamin D.

At two months David had failed to thrive and had persistent candidiasis and diarrhoea. A decision was taken to perform a fetal thymus transplant as soon as a donor became available. The thymus was obtained from a 12-week-old fetus, which was removed as an ectopic tubal pregnancy. The tissue was dissected under sterile conditions and cut into several pieces before being transplanted peritoneally within two hours. A white cell count taken some weeks later showed an increase in cell numbers, but at three months he developed *Pneumocystis carinii* pneumonia, which proved fatal. An autopsy examination confirmed an absent thymus and right sided aortic arch.

QUESTIONS

1 What is the DiGeorge syndrome and how does it affect immune development?
2 What would an immunophenotype of David's lymphocyte population show?
3 To what infections is David especially prone?
4 Is there a chance that future siblings will be affected?
5 Why does David have hypocalcaemia?

NOTES FOR REVISION

YOUR ANSWERS

1 DiGeorge syndrome and how it affects immune development

2 Immunophenotype of David's lymphocyte population

3 Infections to which David is especially prone

4 Chance of future siblings being affected

5 Why David has hypocalcaemia

CASE 7

p. 18.5

ANSWERS

1 DiGeorges syndrome and how it affects immune development

The DiGeorge syndrome is a developmental disorder of the third and fourth pharyngeal pouches. This causes abnormalities of the face and ears, parathyroid insufficiency, congenital heart disease, and thymic hypoplasia or aplasia. It is thymic hypoplasia or aplasia which is responsible for the increased susceptibility to infection.

The thymus is a critical tissue in the development of the immune system. Bone marrow-derived stem cells migrate to the embryonic thymic rudiment and seed the thymus throughout life. It is thought that a very small number of stem cells is capable of providing the entire T cell repertoire. The thymus provides a site for division and differentiation of T cells. It is also responsible for selection of the T cell repertoire, which occurs by positive and negative selection.

2 Immunophenotype of David's lymphocyte population

The lymphocyte profile of a patient with DiGeorge syndrome depends on the degree of thymic hypoplasia. Aplasia will result in a very low T cell count, often combined with normal or raised B cell numbers. More commonly the thymus is extremely small, but with normal architecture. T cell numbers in these patients are low at birth, but have a normal or high CD4:CD8 ratio and recover by the age of five. Severely affected patients are also unable to produce an antibody response to immunisation due to deficient T helper cell activity.

3 Infections to which David is especially prone

Patients with DiGeorge syndrome have an increased susceptibility to a variety of infectious agents. Typically, they can present with recurrent pneumonia (including PCP) and chronic sinusitis caused by *H. influenzae*. Oral candida and persistent diarrhoea are common. Viral infections are frequently caused by herpes simplex and zoster viruses.

4 Chance of future siblings being affected

A few familial clusters have been identified, but the majority of cases appear to be sporadic. The incidence of sub-microscopic deletions of chromosome 22 is believed to be as high as 95% of DiGeorge cases. Interestingly, the familial clusters are also associated with chromosome 22.

5 Why David has hypocalcaemia

The parathyroid glands are also derived from the third and fourth pharyngeal pouches, the third providing the inferior glands and the fourth, the superior. The DiGeorge abnormality is therefore usually complicated by primary hypoparathyroidism manifested as hypocalcaemia, hyperphosphataemia, and low or absent parathyroid hormone.

CASE 8

Mr Doyle, a 51-year-old man, was seen in a respiratory clinic with a three-week history of shortness of breath and a dry cough. Previous episodes of mild chest pain had lead to an initial diagnosis of angina, but he had failed to respond to therapy. On questioning he said his chest pain had subsided and he reported hot flushes. His cough had recently got worse, but there was no sputum or haemoptysis. He did not recall any orthopnoea or peripheral oedema. He was a non-smoker and lived with his male partner with whom he had been having unprotected intercourse for several years. There was no history of intravenous drug use.

On examination Mr Doyle was underweight and afebrile. He had no oedema, but glands were palpable in his cervical, axillary and inguinal regions. His arms, legs and trunk were covered with numerous purple raised cutaneous lesions. A cardiovascular examination was unremarkable. He was tachypnoeic (respiratory rate 25/min) at rest and had mild diffuse crackles across both lung fields. An oral examination showed plaques of *Candida*. The results of investigations are shown in Fig. 3.3.

Fig. 3.3 Results of investigations

Investigation	Result
Haemoglobin	12.8 g/dl
White cell count	Normal
Arterial blood gases PaO_2 $PaCO_2$ pH	9 kPa (normal range 11.3–13.3 kPa) 4.5 kPa (normal range 4.6–6.0 kPa) 7.42 (normal range 7.35–7.45)
Chest radiography	Bilateral diffuse interstitial shadowing
Bronchoscopy with bronchoalveolar lavage	Positive for *Pneumocystis carinii*

Because of his sexual history Mr Doyle was counselled regarding a human immunodeficiency virus (HIV) test and consented. An enzyme-linked immunosorbent assay (ELISA) was positive for anti-HIV antibodies and a polymerase chain reaction (PCR) test directly demonstrated HIV-1. A subsequent differential white cell analysis by flow cytometry showed a depleted CD4$^+$ T cell population with a moderately raised CD8$^+$ cell count. Biopsy of the skin lesions demonstrated Kaposi's sarcoma.

A clear diagnosis of acquired immunodeficiency syndrome (AIDS) was made and Mr Doyle's *Pneumocystis carinii* pneumonia (PCP) was treated with co-trimoxazole. Mr Doyle also agreed to take zidovudine as part of a therapeutic trial. His PCP resolved, but six months later he developed severe pneumonia from which he died shortly afterwards. A post-mortem examination revealed dense consolidation in both lungs and *P. carinii* was isolated.

QUESTIONS

1 What serological markers can be used for the diagnosis and monitoring of HIV infection?

2 What diagnostic tests should be used in suspected HIV infection of a mother and her child infected transplacentally?

3 What is zidovudine and how does it interfere with the HIV life cycle?

4 What effect does HIV infection have on the B cell population?

YOUR ANSWERS

1 Serological markers for the diagnosis and monitoring of HIV infection

2 Diagnostic tests for suspected HIV infection for:
- **a mother**

- **her child infected transplacentally?**

3 What is zidovudine and how does it interfere with the HIV life cycle?

4 What effect does HIV infection have on the B cell population?

CASE 8

pp. 15.7, 18.7

ANSWERS

1 Serological markers for the diagnosis and monitoring of HIV infection

Approximately 95% of HIV-positive individuals seroconvert by three months following infection. ELISA tests for antibodies to Gp120, an HIV surface glycoprotein, and p24, a core protein, can be confirmed by Western blot analysis to eliminate false positive results. Assay of HIV antigen may detect infection before antibody can be detected. Assay of HIV antigen may not be positive because it may be complexed with antibody and not readily measured by immunoassay techniques.

2 Diagnostic tests for suspected HIV infection for:

- **a mother**

The mother's serological state can be tested by ELISA and if necessary confirmed by Western blot.

- **her child infected transplacentally**

There is a problem when assessing the serological status of the baby. Because of transplacental passage of maternal antibody, measurement of the infant's antibody level is not a reliable index of infection because there is maternal IgG specific for HIV in the circulation. For this reason, assessment of the infectious state of the child can only be securely made by PCR, which directly demonstrates the virus. After 18 months of age, serological assessment is more reliable.

3 What is zidovudine and how does it interfere with the HIV life cycle?

Zidovudine is 3'-azido-2',3'-dideoxythymidine. It acts at the stage of production of a DNA copy of the viral RNA. After entry into cells, this is phosphorylated by cellular enzymes to form zidovudine triphosphate, which is an analogue of thymidine triphosphate used in DNA synthesis. It foils viral replication in two ways:

- Firstly, it competes for the active site of reverse transcriptase with functional nucleoside triphosphates (competitive inhibition).
- Secondly, it replaces thymidine triphosphate in a reverse transcribed strand of viral DNA and terminates the chain because it has no hydroxyl group to bind the next nucleoside triphosphate.

4 What effect does HIV infection have on the B cell population?

People with HIV have an increased number of immature B cells with polyclonal activation leading to hypergammaglobulinaemia. There is an increase in IgG1 and IgG3, IgD, and IgA, with IgM and IgE being elevated in children. There is also a reduction of IgG2 and IgG4. The loss of B cell function reflects the disturbance in the CD4 T cell population, but is also due to the direct effect of HIV proteins on B cells.

CASE 9

At 18 months of age Justin developed a swelling in the left inguinal region, which gradually became red and then became an abscess. This discharged pus, which grew *Staphylococcus aureus*. Over the next few months Justin developed episodes of fever and was found to have a bone abscess and microabscesses in his gut wall, which resulted in diarrhoea and obviously prejudiced his nutrition. On two occasions he had a generalised septicaemia, which as with all the other infections was treated with antibiotics. In addition to the *Staph. aureus* infections, Gram-negative organisms and *Aspergillus* were cultured from his infected lesions. Justin has three siblings, all of whom are girls.

In the following three years, Justin was found to have a large liver and spleen and numerous sterile granulomatous lesions in various tissues. He was placed on regular co-trimoxazole, which reduced the frequency of infections reasonably successfully. He was also given white blood cell transfusions during acute infective episodes. Gamma interferon was also tried. His polymorphs were negative in the NBT dye test, but other aspects of function were normal. A diagnosis of chronic granulomatous disease (CGD) was made.

QUESTIONS

1 What is the genetic inheritance of CGD?
2 What is the cell defect?
3 Why are some organisms more frequently the cause of infections, *Staph. aureus* in particular?
4 What other defects may mimic CGD?

NOTES FOR REVISION

YOUR ANSWERS

1 Genetic inheritance of CGD

2 Cell defect of CGD

3 Why some organisms, particularly *Staph. aureus*, are more often the cause of infections

4 Other defects mimicking CGD

CASE 9

pp. 15.14, 18.9–18.10

ANSWERS

1 Genetic inheritance of CGD

Most affected individuals are boys and the inheritance is X-linked recessive. Some cases result from defects in other components in the system and are inherited as autosomal recessive.

2 Cell defect of CGD

The main lesion is failure of NADPH-oxidase; in the inherited group there are lesions in the gene coding for the large beta subunit of the cytochrome-b. One-third are due to recessively inherited defects in the gene encoding p47-phox, p67-phox and p22.

3 Why some organisms, particularly *Staph. aureus,* are more often the cause of infections

The respiratory burst on phagocytosis generates microbiocidal reactive oxygen intermediates (ROI). Patients with CGD cannot kill *Staph. aureus* and certain other bacteria and fungi that are catalase positive because they do not produce peroxide, which would normally kill the microorganisms.

4 Other defects mimicking CGD

Severe G6PD deficiency may mimic CGD because of the greatly decreased production of the substrate NADPH by the pentose phosphate cycle, which may then result in susceptibility to infections.

CASE 10

At 23 years of age, Mrs Dunn suddenly developed a swelling approximately six inches in diameter on her thoracic wall. Her own doctor diagnosed urticaria and prescribed antihistamines. Over 2–3 days the swelling cleared. Six months later she was admitted to hospital with acute abdominal pain and diarrhoea, but a normal white cell count. An abdominal radiograph showed separation of the bowel loops due to mucosal oedema. The symptoms settled without operation. In the following months she had repeated episodes of skin rashes, which were attributed to foods or drugs and were again diagnosed as urticaria. The next occasion led to a marked swelling on her face—acute angioedema. None of the lesions were itchy. The frequency of the episodes increased until she became pregnant and in the last two trimesters these skin symptoms cleared. None of her family had similar symptoms. The results of investigations are shown in Fig. 3.4.

Fig. 3.4 Results of investigations

Investigation	Result
Skin tests	Negative to a range of allergens
Total IgE	Normal
Radioallergosorbent test (RAST)	Negative
Immunoelectophoresis	Normal
Serum proteins	Normal
Liver function tests	Normal
Complement studies C2 and C4 C1 inhibitor (C1INH)	Lower than normal levels Less than 50% of the normal range

A diagnosis of hereditary angioedema (HAE) was made.

QUESTIONS
1 What are the functions of C1 inhibitor?
2 What are the genetics of HAE?
3 What are the *in vitro* differences between the hereditary angioderma and acquired C1 inhibitor deficiency?
4 What treatments are available?

NOTES FOR REVISION

YOUR ANSWERS
1 Functions of C1 inhibitor

2 Genetics of HAE

3 *In vitro* differences between the hereditary and acquired HAE

4 Treatments

CASE 10

pp. 12.5–12.6, 18.8–18.9

ANSWERS

1 Functions of C1 inhibitor

The main function of C1 inhibitor is to block the actions of activated C1. The absence of C1 inhibitor allows the activation of C1 and the generation of C1s and other serine proteases, which C1 inhibitor regulates. The mediators that are then produced lead to the angioedema. Interestingly, if purified C1s is injected into the skin, an intense wheal is produced.

2 Genetics of HAE

HAE is transmitted as an autosomal dominant with high penetrance. This means that the patients are heterozygotes and have one normal gene.

3 *In vitro* differences between the hereditary angioderma and acquired C1 inhibitor deficiency

Both during an attack and during quiescent phases it is likely that the levels of C2 and C4 are low in patients with the hereditary form of the condition, but C1 is normal. In patients with the acquired form, C1 is often depleted. Lymphoproliferative disorders are associated with the acquired form.

4 Treatments

The level of C1INH can be raised by treatments with non-virilising androgens, such as danazol. Inhibition of the activation of the enzymes with which C1INH reacts can also be effective. Compounds such as epsilon amino caproic acid or tranexamic acid can be used. Purified C1INH is now available for intravenous administration.

chapter 4

Type I Hypersensitivity

▨ CASE 11

Mrs Walters, a 69-year-old lady, was admitted to hospital with a community-acquired pneumonia diagnosed by her doctor. She had been admitted before on several occasions with chest infections caused by *Streptococcus pneumoniae*. On arrival she was dehydrated, hypoxic, and confused. Her blood pressure was 120/75 mm Hg and she had a pulse rate of 105 beats/min. A reliable history was not forthcoming and her medical notes were unavailable. The duty doctor decided to treat her with oxygen and intravenous saline and benzylpenicillin, an agent with known activity against *Strep. pneumoniae*.

Several minutes after administering the antibiotics Mrs Walters complained of an itching sensation and cramping abdominal pain. Shortly afterwards she felt faint and became acutely short of breath. Moments later she collapsed and lost consciousness on the ward. The emergency doctor noted that she had swollen eyelids and lips, with patchy erythema across her chest and thighs. She had a cardiac output, but her blood pressure was found to be 70/55 mm Hg. The doctor immediately lowered the head of the bed to maintain cerebral perfusion. He then administered 1 ml of 1/1000 adrenaline intramuscularly and 10 mg of chlorpheniramine (an H1-receptor antagonist) intravenously with 100 mg of hydrocortisone. She regained consciousness and was noted to have a blood pressure of 100/75 mm Hg.

On investigation Mrs Walters was found to have a raised total serum IgE. A radioallergosorbent test (RAST) for benzylpenicillin-specific IgE was strongly positive. Her previous medical notes contained a history of penicillin administration with a resulting episode of erythema and mild urticaria. A diagnosis of anaphylactic shock from benzylpenicillin sensitivity was made. Her pneumonia was successfully treated with vancomycin and she was informed of her drug allergy.

QUESTIONS
1 What was the mechanism of Mrs Walter's anaphylactic shock?
2 Would skin tests have been helpful?
3 Is it possible to desensitise patients to penicillin?
4 What precautions should be taken to ensure that this does not happen again?

NOTES FOR REVISION

YOUR ANSWERS
1 Mechanism of Mrs Walter's anaphylactic shock

2 Use of skin tests

3 Is it possible to desensitise patients to penicillin?

4 Precautions to ensure that this does not happen again

CASE 11

pp. 19.2–19.3, 19.14

ANSWERS

1 Mechanism of Mrs Walter's anaphylactic shock
This is a typical Type I hypersensitivity reaction. In this case the absorbed penicillin is bound by IgE on basophils and possibly mast cells, leading to intravascular histamine release and anaphylactic shock. The released histamine leads to capillary dilatation and a fall in blood pressure.

2 Use of skin tests
Skin tests can be helpful for Type I hyersensitivity, but have to be done with great care. A useful preparation for penicillin allergy is penicilloyl polylysine. Skin prick tests should be done with great care being exercised before any drug is given intradermally.

3 Is it possible to desensitise patients to penicillin?
Desensitisation has been attempted and in some cases successfully, but is not generally recommended.

4 Precautions to ensure that this does not happen again
Mrs Walters' hospital notes and those of her family doctor should have the information very clearly noted, preferably on the outside of the notes and in large letters. Mrs Walters should also wear at all times a bracelet or necklace clearly stating details of her allergy.

CASE 12

Mrs Young, a 62-year-old lady, was stung by a bee from a hive in her back garden. Harvesting the honey had left her with several stings during the course of the summer. Several minutes after being stung she complained of an itching sensation and cramping abdominal pain. Shortly afterwards she felt faint and acutely short of breath. Moments later she collapsed and lost consciousness. Her husband, a doctor, noticed that her breathing was rapid and wheezy and that she had swollen eyelids and lips. She was pale and had patchy erythema across her neck and arms.

On examination her apex beat could be felt, but her radial pulse was weak. Her husband immediately administered 0.5 ml of 1/1000 adrenaline intramuscularly and 10 mg of chlorpheniramine (an H1-receptor antihistamine) intravenously with 100 mg of hydrocortisone. She regained consciousness and her respiratory rate dropped. By the following day she had recovered completely.

On investigation Mrs Young was found to have a raised total serum IgE. A radioallergosorbent test (RAST) for bee venom-specific IgE was strongly positive; a similar test for wasp venom was negative. A diagnosis of anaphylactic shock due to bee venom sensitivity was made and a decision taken to commence desensitisation therapy.

Mrs Young was made aware of the possible risk of the procedure and consented to it. She was injected subcutaneously with gradually increasing doses of bee venom, the procedures being performed in hospital with access to resuscitation apparatus. No further allergic reactions occurred and she was maintained on a dose of bee venom at one-month intervals for the next two years. She was stung by a bee the following summer and had no adverse reaction.

QUESTIONS

1 How can you determine whether or not a patient is allergic to bee venom?
2 What is the mechanism involved in the anaphylactic response?
3 Can someone without specific IgE antibodies to bee venom have an anaphylactic reaction following a sting?
4 Desensitisation is very effective. What is the mechanism of protection?

NOTES FOR REVISION

YOUR ANSWERS

1 How to determine whether or not a patient is allergic to bee venom

2 Mechanism involved in the anaphylactic response

3 Can someone without specific IgE antibodies to bee venom have an anaphylactic reaction following a sting?

4 Mechanism of protection due to desensitisation

CASE 12

pp. 19.2–19.3, 25.6

ANSWERS

1 How to determine whether or not a patient is allergic to bee venom

The patient must give a relevant history of an anaphylactic reaction to a defined sting first. RAST is very useful and if high is strongly supportive of the diagnosis. Quantitative end-point skin testing will give an estimate of the patient's sensitivity.

2 Mechanism involved in the anaphylactic response

The anaphylactic reaction is a typical Type I hypersensitivity reaction involving histamine release from mast cells and basophils.

3 Can someone without specific IgE antibodies to bee venom have an anaphylactic reaction following a sting?

One of the major venom allergens is mellitin and this can activate the alternative pathway of complement, thereby producing C3a and C5a. These, as anaphylatoxins can release histamine from mast cells, thus mimicking exactly an IgE-mediated Type I reaction in the absence of specific IgE.

4 Mechanism of protection due to desensitisation

The mechanism of protection is not exactly understood, but probably reflects the production of blocking IgG antibodies. These then compete for the venom and block access to IgE on mast cells.

CASE 13

Jennifer, a nine-year-old girl, was seen by her doctor with a three-month history of coughing, wheezy breathing, and insomnia. Recently, she had become extremely breathless after helping her mother to clean the house. She had no previous history of prolonged respiratory tract infections. Childhood illnesses had included measles, mumps, and atopic eczema, which had proved refractory to topical emollient and corticosteroid therapy. Her mother had also had atopic eczema up to adolescence and suffered from allergic rhinitis.

On examination Jennifer was on the 50th centile for height and weight. She had no finger clubbing and was not tachycardic or febrile. She was not tachypnoeic at rest, had good chest expansion, and resonant lung fields to percussion. On auscultation she had a mild expiratory wheeze in both lung fields. A cardiovascular examination was unremarkable. The results of investigations are shown in Fig. 4.1.

Fig. 4.1 Results of investigations

Investigation	Result
Peak expiratory flow rate	Below normal range for height and age
Haemoglobin	Normal
White cell count	Raised
Differential white cell analysis	Eosinophilia
Total serum IgE	Elevated
Skin prick test	Positive for house dust mite, grass, and cat
Sputum examination	Large quantities of green mucoid plugs and eosinophils

A diagnosis of allergic (extrinsic) asthma was made. Her doctor advised her to avoid contact with dust and her pet cat and to buy a protective sheet for her mattress. An inhaled dose of salbutamol, a beta-2 receptor agonist, produced an increase in the peak expiratory flow rate and resolved her cough. She was prescribed a short course of systemic corticosteroids and an inhaler containing sodium cromoglycate (Intal, Cromogen), a prophylactic drug believed to prevent mast cell inflammatory mediator release. The combination of the two drugs was sufficient to control her asthma, which resolved by the age of 22.

QUESTIONS

1 What is the mechanism of allergic asthma?
2 What is the cause of the late-phase reaction?
3 Are basophils implicated in the inflammatory process?
4 Can beta agonists make the patient more sensitive to allergen exposure?
5 What are the chances of this patient having allergic children?

NOTES FOR REVISION

YOUR ANSWERS

1 Mechanism of allergic asthma

2 Cause of the late-phase reaction

3 Are basophils implicated in the inflammatory process?

4 Can beta agonists make the patient more sensitive to allergen exposure?

5 Chances of this patient having allergic children

CASE 13

pp. 19.3, 19.15–19.17

ANSWERS

1 Mechanism of allergic asthma

The initial reaction in allergic asthma is allergen triggering IgE on mast cells in the lung to release histamine and other mediators. Following this acute reaction there is a late-phase reaction up to 12 hours later with cell infiltration and a further fall in lung function. The initial and late phase reactions are blocked by sodium cromoglycate and the late phase by corticosteroids. It is the late-phase reaction (LPR) that causes the chronic inflammatory response in the lungs.

2 Cause of the late-phase reaction

The LPR is dependent on triggering of the immediate Type I response. Various inflammatory mediators and cytokines are released and lead to secondary inflammation with a cellular infiltration. This complex cascade leads to broncial hyperreactivity.

3 Are basophils implicated in the inflammatory process?

Certainly in the nose the mediators released in the LPR are those of the basophil. Adhesion molecules, especially VCAM which is induced by IL-4, preferentially bind eosinophils and basophils.

4 Can beta agonists make the patient more sensitive to allergen exposure?

There are data that show that after treatment with beta agonists the dose of allergen needed to produce a given fall in lung function is less than when such drugs are not given. The response to other spasmogens is unchanged.

5 Chances of this patient having allergic children

The genetics of atopy is not clearly defined. However, allergic parents have more allergic children than those who are not. If one parent is allergic, approximately 30% of the children will be atopic, and this percentage doubles if both parents are allergic.

chapter 5

Type II Hypersensitivity

 CASE 14

Simon, a 10-year-old schoolboy, was seen by his doctor with a three-week history of polyuria, excessive thirst, and a weight loss of two kilos. Childhood illnesses had included mumps and measles, which resolved without incident. His brother aged seven was fit and well, but there was a family history of thyroiditis and pernicious anaemia.

On examination Simon was underweight for his height and age. Respiratory, cardiovascular, and abdominal examinations were unremarkable. The results of investigations are shown in Fig. 5.1.

Fig. 5.1 Results of investigations

Investigation	Result
White cell count	Normal
Haemoglobin	Normal
Urinalysis	Glycosuria
Two consecutive random blood glucose tests	Above 10 mmol/l
Renal function (estimated by serum urea and creatinine levels)	Normal
Circulating pancreatic islet cell antibodies	Positive by indirect immunofluorescence

A diagnosis of insulin-dependent diabetes mellitus (IDDM) was made. Further tests were performed to eliminate the possibility of other organ-specific auto-immune diseases in the light of an extensive family history. Thyroid function tests were normal and he had no evidence of autoantibodies to thyroid antigens or intrinsic factor. He was given advice about modifying his diet and was started on subcutaneous injections of insulin to normalise his blood glucose level. At routine follow-up he was coping well with the regimen and had a well-controlled blood glucose level.

QUESTIONS
1 What is the classification of diabetes mellitus?
2 What is the immunopathology of IDDM?
3 What are the genetics of IDDM?
4 What is the chance of immunotherapy stopping the disease process?

NOTES FOR REVISION

YOUR ANSWERS

1 Classification of diabetes mellitus

2 Immunopathology of IDDM

3 Genetics of IDDM

4 Chance of immunotherapy stopping the disease process

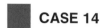 **CASE 14**

pp. 8.12, 9.12–9.14

ANSWERS

1 Classification of diabetes mellitus

Diabetes has been classified according to whether patients treated successfully are dependent (Type I–IDDM) or non-dependent (Type II–NIDDM) on insulin. Type I occurs more frequently in younger subjects and is characterised by the typical diabetic symptoms. Type II occurs in a group of older patients, often overweight (85%), who present insidiously.

2 Immunopathology of IDDM

In spite of the acute onset, the diabetes is the result of a long latent period during which the islets have become progressively damaged. This period is characterised by the loss of the first phase of insulin response to intravenous glucose and by the presence of islet cell antibodies (ICA). The islets are infiltrated by lymphocytes, reflecting a cellular response to an autoantigen. The islet cell antibody is an organ-specific antibody that is present in 70–80% of patients at diagnosis, but tends to disappear afterwards, presumably associated with the loss of antigenic stimulus when the islet number is reduced.

3 Genetics of IDDM

Susceptibility to the disease is thought to be part environmental and part genetic, but to involve multiple genes. There is good evidence that genes in the HLA-D region of the short arm of chromosome 6 confer susceptibility to IDDM. About 95% of Caucasians with IDDM have HLA-DR3 or DR4 or both genes compared with 50% in the general population. There may be an even closer link with a DQ locus.

4 Chance of immunotherapy stopping the disease process

IDDM is immunologically mediated and attempts to stop islet cell destruction with immunosuppressive agents are likely to fail, as even at the time of diagnosis, islet cell destruction has been proceeding for a long time. Cyclosporin A has been given to newly diagnosed insulin-requiring diabetics, and a proportion (25%) have been retained in remission for up to a year. There might be a problem with long-term treatment with this drug in spite of this obvious benefit.

CASE 15

Mr Edwards, a 28-year-old dry cleaner, presented in A&E with a two-week history of malaise, dizziness, nausea, and 'puffy eyes'. He had also noticed that despite a normal fluid intake he was emptying his bladder less frequently than normal. On direct questioning he had no symptoms relating to the respiratory system and had no family history of disease. He smoked 20 cigarettes a day.

On examination Mr Edwards had diffuse oedema, especially periorbitally, and his blood pressure was 150/110 mm Hg. He also had a low-grade fever. The rest of his cardiovascular and respiratory examination was normal and he had no rashes or joint pain. The results of investigations are shown in Fig. 5.2.

Fig. 5.2 Results of investigations

Investigation	Result
Urinalysis	Microscopic haematuria, proteinuria, and granular casts
Haemoglobin	Unusually low considering the duration and nature of the symptoms
Renal ultrasound scanning and cystoscopy	No cause for haematuria identified

While staying in hospital Mr Edwards' serum urea and creatinine rose, indicating a deterioration in renal function. His urine output decreased and his proteinuria and haematuria persisted. A renal biopsy revealed glomerular lesions consisting of a proliferation of both epithelial and mesangial cells. Crescent formation was also visible in part of the sample. A diagnosis of crescentic glomerulonephritis was made and further tests performed to elucidate the cause.

Complement levels were normal, thus excluding systemic lupus erythematosus with renal impairment. Blood cultures were negative and there was no history of a streptococcal infection. Furthermore, there was an absence of circulating immune complexes, eliminating a post-streptococcal cause. Further analysis of the biopsy specimen using fluorescence microscopy showed a linear deposition of IgG along the glomerular basement membrane. An enzyme-linked immuno-sorbent assay (ELISA) performed on Mr Edwards' serum demonstrated anti-glomerular basement membrane (GBM) antibodies. A diagnosis of Goodpasture's syndrome was made. A subsequent chest radiograph showed interstitial shadowing, and this, combined with an unusually low haemoglobin level, suggested lung haemorrhage initiated by the antibodies.

Mr Edwards was prescribed a course of corticosteroids and cyclophosphamide. This was combined with plasmapheresis to remove anti-GBM antibodies and renal dialysis to supplement poor renal function. Levels of circulating anti-GBM antibody dropped steadily over the six-week treatment period and there was a corresponding improvement in renal function. While convalescing on the ward, the area around his arteriovenous shunt became infected. He concurrently developed a cough with haemoptysis associated with a rise in serum urea and creatinine levels. Anti-GBM antibodies were found to be raised. Treatment was restarted and antibiotics were added to clear his local *Staphylococcus aureus* infection. His subsequent progress was good and he was discharged from hospital.

QUESTIONS

1 What is the picture seen on immunofluorescence when the patient's serum is overlaid on a section of normal lung or kidney and subsequently stained with a conjugated anti-immunoglobulin?
2 What is the mechanism of damage to the lung and kidney?
3 Is plasmapheresis curative?
4 Why did the skin infection at the site of the arteriovenous shunt precipitate a further episode of disease?

YOUR ANSWERS

1 Picture on immunofluorescence

2 Mechanism of damage to the lung and kidney

3 Is plasmapheresis curative?

4 Why the skin infection precipitated a further episode of disease

CASE 15

pp. 12.6, 20.10–20.11, 24.6, Fig 21.3

ANSWERS

1 Picture on immunofluorescence

The picture seen on immunofluorescence is a smooth labelling of the antibody over the surface of the lung alveolus or glomerular basement membrane. This is to be contrasted with the punctate staining which is found where there is deposition of immune complexes of antibody and antigen, typical of Type III hypersensitivity.

2 Mechanism of damage to the lung and kidney

This is a typical Type II hypersensitivity reaction where antibody is bound to an antigen associated with a cell surface or membrane, complement is fixed, and local damage occurs through that activation, made worse by cell accumulation.

3 Is plasmapheresis curative?

The antibody directed against the glomerular basement membrane and the alveolar basement membrane is the 'cause' of the inflammation. In this condition plasmapheresis together with immunosuppressive drugs can indeed be a 'cure' in that the inflammatory process can resolve. If the damage to the glomeruli is not end stage, some recovery can take place. This must be one of the few autoimmune conditions that can be relieved by removing antibody from the circulation.

4 Why the skin infection precipitated a further episode of disease

It is difficult to give an exact explanation of this phenomenon. It is likely that there was still antibody in the circulation. The infection in the arteriovenous shunt must have lead to the production of inflammatory mediators, which allowed the deposition of the antibody onto the target antigen, reproducing the disease. Treatment with antibiotics and further plasmapheresis is the treatment to be given.

CASE 16

Mrs Lake, a 30-year-old gravida 4 para 1+² lady, was seen at an antenatal booking clinic when five weeks pregnant. Her first pregnancy had been uneventful with the child, a boy, now in his teens. Her second and third pregnancies had resulted in a stillbirth at 32 weeks and a spontaneous abortion at 22 weeks, respectively. She was unaware of any reasons for the lost pregnancies and had subsequently moved from Nigeria to the UK. She had no other medical history of note.

Examination revealed no abnormalities and samples were taken for blood grouping and rubella status. The results of these tests and those for her husband are shown in Fig. 5.3.

Fig. 5.3 Results of investigations

Investigation	Result
Mrs Lake	
Blood group	A positive; Rhesus-D-negative (cde/cde)
Anti-D antibody	7 i.u./ml
Rubella antibody	Negative
Husband	
Blood group	A positive, Rh-D-positive (CDe/CDe)

These results implied that the fetus was heterozygous for the D antigen and therefore D positive (CDe/cde). As Mrs Lake was also rubella antibody negative she was advised to seek immunisation in the puerperium.

Mrs Lake's history and rhesus status were an indication for monitoring maternal anti-D levels and fetal haemoglobin throughout the pregnancy to prevent haemolytic disease of the newborn (HDN). Serum samples taken for analysis at three-week intervals showed a rise in anti-D levels to 10 i.u./ml at 17 weeks. Amniocentesis was performed, which yielded a sample for spectroscopic estimation of bile pigments. Severe haemolysis was demonstrated and intrauterine transfusion of the fetus was carried out using fresh (less than seven days old) Rh D-negative blood. Further fetal blood evaluation by fetoscopy showed continuing anaemia, which was corrected with three more transfusions before delivery.

Continuing risk to the child was an indication for elective Caesarean section at 34 weeks. A live male infant was delivered with signs of jaundice and anaemia. Cord blood samples confirmed that the child was Rh D-positive and anaemic, with a raised serum bilirubin. Exchange transfusion of 500 ml of Rh D-negative blood ABO-matched to the child was performed to alleviate the anaemia and phototherapy was used to degrade the bilirubin. One further transfusion was required, but the child then made an uneventful recovery.

QUESTIONS

1 What is the mechanism of this disease process?
2 For every 20 Rhesus-incompatible pregnancies only one or two may develop HDN. Why?
3 What is the rationale for administering anti-D antibodies to the mother?
4 Why is the incidence of ABO HDN much lower than the rate of incompatibility?

NOTES FOR REVISION

YOUR ANSWERS

1 **Mechanism of rhesus incompatibility**

2 **Why only a minority of Rhesus-incompatible pregnancies develop HDN**

3 **Rationale for administering anti-D antibodies to the mother**

4 **Why the incidence of ABO HDN is much lower than the rate of incompatibility**

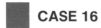 **CASE 16**

pp. 20.6–20.7

ANSWERS

1 Mechanism of Rhesus incompatibility

Destruction of fetal red blood cells can occur when maternal IgG specific for red cell epitopes crosses the placenta. The cells become coated by the antibody and are destroyed by the fetal phagocytic system. The antibodies may be raised against either the ABO or Rhesus antigens. Sensitisation occurs when the mother is exposed to fetal red cells following a transplacental haemorrhage or during parturition.

In the case of Rhesus antigens the child is at risk if the mother is Rh D-negative (cde/cde) and the fetus D-positive. Initial maternal exposure to fetal red cells causes a primary antibody response, which often occurs at birth. The first child is therefore not usually affected, although prolonged exposure to fetal cells during pregnancy may rarely cause HDN in a first child. Subsequent Rh D-positive children are at risk from the antibodies because they are of the IgG class and so cross the placenta freely. Haemolysis can cause death by hydrops fetalis (severe fetal oedema) *in utero*. Alternatively the baby can be hypoxic *in utero* or present with symptoms of anaemia and jaundice at birth.

2 Why only a minority of Rhesus-incompatible pregnancies develop HDN

It is believed that many mothers do not become sensitised to the D antigen because of maternal/fetal ABO incompatibility. If such an incompatibility exists then fetal red cells entering the maternal circulation will be coated with antibody and destroyed before they have a chance to provoke a D-antigen specific antibody response. Anti-ABO antibodies are present despite the absence of any exposure to incompatible cells and are believed to arise from cross-sensitisation with bacterial antigens.

3 Rationale for administering anti-D antibodies to the mother

Anti-D antibodies are administered to Rh D-negative women immediately after birth of a Rh D-positive child. Although the precise mechanism of action is not known it is believed that the antibodies coat the D-positive cells and mediate their removal before they can stimulate an endogenous antibody response. The effectiveness of the procedure is demonstrated by the dramatic fall in HDN deaths following the introduction of anti-D prophylaxis in the UK. Anti-D antibodies should also be given after any procedure that might produce a transplacental bleed, such as amniocentesis.

4 Why the incidence of ABO HDN is much lower than the rate of incompatibility

Some 20% of pregnancies are associated with a maternal/fetal ABO incompatibility, but the incidence of HDN is only a fraction of this number. Group A and group B mothers have anti-B and anti-A antibodies, respectively, but they are usually of the IgM class and therefore do not cross the placenta. The majority of ABO HDN occurs with group O mothers who have an increased incidence of IgG anti-B and anti-A antibodies. Most babies with ABO HDN are not profoundly anaemic and less than 0.05% require exchange transfusions.

CASE 17

A 65-year-old man, Mr Brown, presented to his doctor in winter with cold extremities and malaise. His symptoms had been present for several years and always occurred in cold weather. Most recently he had noticed that his urine had been unusually dark, especially when the temperature was low. He was not diabetic, and was a non-smoker and a moderate drinker.

On examination Mr Brown was mildly jaundiced and had an area of acrocyanosis (purple discoloration) at the tip of his nose. His nail beds and sclera were pale. His hands and feet were pale and felt cold, but peripheral pulses were present. When asked he said he had not experienced any pain in his calves. There was no evidence of ulceration and sensation was normal. His liver was not palpable, but his spleen could be felt 1 cm below the costal margin. The rest of his cardiovascular and respiratory examination was normal and he had no chronic stigmata of liver disease. The results of investigations are shown in Fig. 5.4.

Fig. 5.4 Results of investigations

Investigation	Result
Haemoglobin	Below normal range
Blood film produced at room temperature	Marked red cell agglutination, mild spherocytosis and reticulocytosis
Direct antiglobulin test (DAT)	Positive for complement (C3) only on the red cell surface
Serum bilirubin	Elevated
Urobilinogen	Elevated
Haemoglobinuria	Present
Serum IgG and IgA levels	Normal
IgM level	Raised
Antibodies with specificity for the 'I' red cell antigen	Found to react best at 4°C, monoclonal, and of the IgM class
Vitamin B$_{12}$ and folate levels	Normal
White cell count	Normal
Liver function tests	Normal

A diagnosis of cold haemagglutinin disease (CHAD) with autoimmune haemolytic anaemia (AIHA), hyperbilirubinaemia, and Raynaud's phenomenon was made.

QUESTIONS

1 What is the significance of the direct antiglobulin test (DAT) ?
2 What are the causes of CHAD ?
3 How does cold autoimmune haemolytic disease (AIHA) differ from warm AIHA?
4 What treatment should be advised for CHAD ?

NOTES FOR REVISION

YOUR ANSWERS

1 Significance of DAT

2 Causes of CHAD

3 How cold AIHA differs from warm AIHA

4 Treatment for CHAD

CASE 17

p. 20.7

ANSWERS

1 Significance of DAT

The DAT is used to detect antibody and/or complement on the surface of red blood cells that have become bound *in vivo*. The antiglobulin reagent, which consists of a mixture of anti-IgG and anti-complement antibodies, is added to a sample of washed red cells derived from the patient. Agglutination of the cells is a positive result. Examples of conditions that are DAT positive include haemolytic disease of the newborn, autoimmune haemolytic anaemia, and haemolytic transfusion reactions.

2 Causes of CHAD

Cold autoimmune haemolytic anaemia can be either primary (55% of cases) or secondary in origin. The latter can occur following a *Mycoplasma pneumoniae* infection or after an Epstein–Barr virus infection known as infectious mononucleosis (glandular fever). Other causes include malignancies such as chronic lymphocytic leukaemia and non-Hodgkin's lymphoma, as well as rheumatic disorders such as systemic lupus erythematosus and rheumatoid arthritis. Primary cases and those associated with malignancy involve monoclonal antibodies with the remainder being polyclonal.

3 How cold AIHA differs from warm AIHA

See Fig. 5.5.

Fig. 5.5 How cold AIHA differs from warm AIHA

Feature	Warm AIHA	Cold AIHA
Age of patient	30+	60+
Mechanism behind presenting symptoms	Haemolysis	Haemolysis and Raynaud's phenomenon
Cause of anaemia	Opsonisation and phagocytosis	Intravascular haemolysis
Class of antibody	IgG	IgM
Type of Ig response	Polyclonal	Monoclonal/polyclonal
Antibody specificity	Rh antigen	I antigen

4 Treatment for CHAD

Primary treatment is to keep warm and this often improves symptoms. Thereafter alkylating agents such as chlorambucil may be helpful.

CASE 18

Miss Todd, aged 24, began to feel more and more tired despite having a sedentary job with no stress. She complained of muscle tiredness, which became worse with repetitive movements and went to her doctor for tests. He could find no abnormality on general examination and none of her blood tests showed any abnormality. Some weeks later she returned to her doctor having had some episodes of double vision. On this occasion the doctor noted that she had unilateral ptosis and difficulty in opening her hands after making a tight fist.

He injected Tensilon and within minutes her muscle weakness had improved. Tensilon is a drug that blocks acetylcholine esterase and therefore increases the amount of acetylcholine available. Thus a diagnosis of myasthenia gravis was made. Further tests showed the presence of autoantibodies to acetylcholine receptor (AChR) and also to thyroid microsomes. A CT scan of the mediastinum revealed a thymoma.

QUESTIONS
1 What is the mechanism of damage in myasthenia gravis?
2 What are the HLA associations of the disease?
3 Can drug reactions produce a myasthenic condition?
4 What is the diagnostic value of AChR antibodies?

NOTES FOR REVISION

YOUR ANSWERS
1 Mechanism of damage

2 HLA associations

3 Can drug reactions produce a myasthenic condition?

4 Diagnostic value of AChR antibodies?

CASE 18

pp. 12.16, 20.11

ANSWERS

1 Mechanism of damage

Antibody directed against the end plate on the muscle can fix complement and cause direct cell damage. This is a Type II hypersensitivity reaction, which leads to muscle end plate damage and a reduction in the number of acetylcholine receptors. Treatment is primarily aimed at increasing the available acetylcholine by inhibiting acetylcholine esterase.

2 HLA associations

The association of myasthenia gravis with particular immune response genes is influenced by race. In Caucasoids, HLA associations have shown three subgroups:

- Young onset, no thymoma: a strong association with HLA A1, B8, and DR3.
- Old onset, no thymoma: some association with B7 and DR2.
- Thymoma: no obvious association.

3 Can drug reactions produce a myasthenic condition?

It is well recognised that penicillamine, especially in patients with rheumatoid arthritis, can lead to myasthenic symptoms and anti-AChR antibodies. Symptomatic treatment with choline esterase inhibitors is effective, but the disease does remit when the penicillamine is stopped. The anti-AChR antibodies also decrease following withdrawal of the drug.

4 Diagnostic value of acetylcholine receptor antibodies?

Antibodies specific for the AChR have been found in 90% of patients with myasthenia gravis. The titre of antibody and the severity of the disease do not correlate exactly. The majority of patients showing prolonged improvement have a greater than 50% decrease in anti-AChR antibody concentration with time, regardless of the type of treatment.

chapter 6

Type III Hypersensitivity

 CASE 19

Mr Franks, a 55-year-old farm worker, visited his doctor complaining of increasing breathlessness over the previous nine months accompanied by a dry cough, which occurred predominantly at night. He had not experienced any chest pain and had been a lifelong non-smoker. He had no previous history of lung complaints and no family history of cardiovascular disease. He had been in his present job for ten years and considered himself to be physically fit.

On examination Mr Franks had reduced chest expansion bilaterally and marked inspiratory crackles and squeaks on auscultation of his lungs. He had no finger clubbing or palpable lymph nodes. His cardiovascular examination was unremarkable. A simple test using a peak flow meter showed a reduced peak expiratory flow rate. A full blood count was normal and a Mantoux test negative. His doctor referred him to a respiratory unit for further evaluation.

Lung function tests showed a decrease in total lung capacity, vital capacity, and functional residual capacity, and a flow volume curve demonstrated a restrictive defect. A chest radiograph showed bilateral linear and nodular shadowing in the upper and middle zones. A diagnosis of pulmonary fibrosis was made and further tests were carried out to identify the cause. The results of these tests are shown in Fig. 6.1.

Fig. 6.1 Results of further investigations

Investigation	Result
Test for precipitating antibodies with affinity for antigens derived from *Micropolyspora faeni*	Positive
Intradermal injection of *M. faeni* antigens	Positive Arthus reaction at six hours
Bronchoalveolar lavage (BAL)	Increased lymphocytes; CD4$^+$:CD8$^+$ ratio of the T cell population reversed compared with normals
Lung biopsy	Granulomatous lesions centred in the bronchioles

A diagnosis of extrinsic allergic alveolitis (EAA) was made. In this case Mr Franks had inhaled actinomycetes that were growing on stored damp crops. This disease variant is therefore known as Farmer's lung. Management consisted primarily of allergen avoidance using suitable respiratory apparatus. Oral corticosteroids were also administered to reduce the parenchymal inflammation of the lungs.

QUESTIONS

1 Are the precipitating antibodies characteristic of the disease?
2 What is the mechanism of lung damage?
3 Is pulmonary fibrosis likely to continue when the patient is removed from exposure to the antigen?
4 Does cigarette smoking have an effect on the course of the disease?

YOUR ANSWERS

1 Are the precipitating antibodies characteristic of the disease?

2 Mechanism of lung damage

3 Is pulmonary fibrosis likely to continue on removal from exposure to the antigen?

4 Does cigarette smoking have an effect on the course of the disease?

CASE 19

pp. 21.2, 21.4

ANSWERS

1 Are the precipitating antibodies characteristic of the disease?

High levels of IgG antibody are present in this condition and precipitation in agar gel is characteristic of EAA. However, some exposed farmers do have precipitins, but are asymptomatic. This suggests that there are other factors that lead to the lung damage.

2 Mechanism of lung damage

In the presence of high levels of IgG antibody, inhaled allergen forms immune complexes in the lung parenchyma and leads to a Type III reaction with complement fixation and subsequent local damage associated with cell infiltration.

3 Is pulmonary fibrosis likely to continue on removal from exposure to the antigen?

In some patients lung fibrosis continues even when exposure has stopped. The mechanism is unknown.

4 Does cigarette smoking have an effect on the course of the disease?

In Farmer's lung and Bird Fancier's lung, the relevant precipitating antibodies are more common in non-smokers than smokers. The reason for this is not known, but it may reflect an impairment of alveolar macrophage phagocytosis and antigen presentation in tobacco smokers. This cannot be taken as a recommendation to smoke cigarettes!

CASE 20

At the end of a trip abroad, Yvonne, aged 35, developed acute diarrhoea and some vomiting. On her return home she visited her doctor who gave her an antibiotic co-trimoxazole (sulphamethoxazole and trimethoprim), which she was to take for eight days. She finished the course and three days later developed some red itchy lumps on her skin and a headache. This was associated with aching and swollen joints, mainly wrists and knees although her hands were also affected. The headache was not severe, but she decided to visit her doctor.

Yvonne's doctor confirmed that her rash was urticaria and that her joints were swollen. Her temperature was also raised. Examination of her urine showed evidence of protein, and a full blood count was normal with only a minimal elevation of the eosinophil count. He gave Yvonne antihistamines and told her that the rash and joint swelling would clear in a few days. A diagnosis of drug allergy was made.

QUESTIONS

1 What is the likely mechanism of the reaction?
2 Is it made less likely because the rash appeared after she had stopped taking the antibiotic?
3 Would any blood test be helpful?
4 Can Yvonne take this antibiotic again safely in six months' time?

NOTES FOR REVISION

YOUR ANSWERS

1 Likely mechanism of the reaction

2 Is this mechanism made less likely because the rash appeared after she had stopped taking the antibiotic?

3 Would any blood test be helpful?

4 Can Yvonne take this antibiotic again safely in six months' time?

CASE 20

pp. 21.4

ANSWERS

1 Likely mechanism of the reaction

The mechanism is likely to be a serum sickness reaction with immune complexes leading to the systemic symptomatology. The complexes of drug and antibody (IgG) will deposit in various tissues, fix complement and cause an inflammatory response; thus the widespread symptoms.

2 Is this mechanism made less likely because the rash appeared after Yvonne had stopped taking the antibiotic?

If the reaction is due to immune complexes, it is possible that when the drug concentration in the blood fell when the tablets were stopped, immune complex formation could take place in optimal proportions and thus allow 'precipitation' in the body.

3 Would any blood test be helpful?

Probably not, although the detection of immune complexes might have given some weight to the diagnosis. Immune complex assays are notoriously difficult and are not used routinely in diagnostic laboratories now.

4 Can Yvonne take this antibiotic again safely in six months' time?

No, she should not take this mixture again. It is likely that the sulpha-methoxazole was the cause. She could try trimethoprim on a future occasion and it might not cause a reaction, but giving a different family of antibiotics would be wiser.

CASE 21

Mr Jackson, a 31-year-old Irishman, presented to his doctor with a six-month history of malaise, anorexia, weight loss, mild diffuse abdominal pain and diarrhoea, and the recent development of an itchy blistering rash on the extensor surfaces of his knees and elbows. He had also vomited two to three times a week for the previous fortnight. He had no history of foreign travel. His family lived in Ireland and he had no past history of ill health.

On examination Mr Jackson had finger clubbing, several aphthous mouth ulcers, and angular cheilitis. He was not oedematous and had no signs of anaemia. Examination of his cardiovascular and respiratory systems was unremarkable. He had a mildly distended abdomen, which was not tender. No masses were felt on palpation or on rectal examination. Mr Jackson's doctor decided to refer him to a gastroenterologist for further evaluation.

In the clinic, Mr Jackson's skin rash was identified as dermatitis herpetiformis. The results of investigations are shown in Fig. 6.2.

Fig. 6.2 Results of investigations

Investigation	Result
Blood film	Macrocytic anaemia and presence of Howell–Jolly bodies (found in patients with hyposplenism)
Serum folate and red cell folate	Below normal range
Serum iron values	Below normal range
White cell count	Normal
Platelet count	Normal
Serum IgM, IgG, and IgE	Normal
Serum IgA	Elevated
Urea and creatinine	Normal
Electrolyte analysis	Mild hypomagnesaemia and hypocalcaemia
Parathyroid hormone	High
Serum albumin	Low

Mr Jackson had evidence of both folate and iron deficiency anaemia, and also mild secondary hyperparathyroidism.

A working diagnosis of coeliac disease (gluten enteropathy) was made and a jejunal biopsy performed. The presence of subtotal villous atrophy, elongated crypts and a dense inflammatory infiltrate were strongly suggestive of coeliac disease. Enzyme-linked immunosorbent assay (ELISA) demonstrated abnormally high levels of serum antibodies to alpha-gliadin with high titres also to reticulin.

Mr Jackson saw a dietitian who outlined a gluten-free diet and provided calcium, folate, and iron supplements. He gained several kilos in weight over the next six months and his symptoms improved considerably. Anti-alpha-gliadin and reticulin antibody levels performed at a follow-up visit were lower than those at presentation. A repeat jejunal biopsy showed an improvement in the architecture. Mr Jackson was advised to observe a gluten-free diet for the rest of his life. Regular follow-up appointments were arranged because of the increased risk of small bowel malignancy in patients with coeliac disease.

QUESTIONS

1 What is the connection between dermatitis herpetiformis and coeliac disease?
2 Are antibody determinations sufficient to make the diagnosis of coeliac disease?
3 Can other foods cause the same clinical picture?
4 Is it really necessary to avoid gluten for life?

YOUR ANSWERS

1 Connection between dermatitis herpetiformis and coeliac disease

2 Are antibody determinations sufficient to diagnose coeliac disease?

3 Can other foods cause the same clinical picture?

4 Is it really necessary to avoid gluten for life?

CASE 21

p. 21.1

ANSWERS

1 Connection between dermatitis herpetiformis and coeliac disease
More than 95% of patients with dermatitis herpetiformis (DH) have an abnormal jejunal mucosa. The lesion is patchy and responds to a gluten-free diet. Dapsone suppresses the skin lesions, possibly by blocking the release of neutrophil chemotactic factors. The mechanism of DH is probably the deposition of immune complexes, especially as IgA can be seen as granular deposits in the subepidermal region.

2 Are antibody determinations sufficient to diagnose coeliac disease?
Levels of antigliadin antibodies can be a help in making the diagnosis and can be used in monitoring compliance in adhering to the gluten-free diet. Reticulin antibodies can also be a useful marker for diagnosis. The gold standard for diagnosis is the jejunal biopsy and of course the response to diet.

3 Can other foods cause the same clinical picture?
Other foods have been implicated in gastrointestinal villous atrophy: for example, eggs, milk, and chicken. It is thought that this is not such a long lasting or severe syndrome.

4 Is it really necessary to avoid gluten for life?
The exact immunopathological mechanism in coeliac disease is not clear. What is clear is that gluten taken after many years of abstention still causes mucosal damage. It is for this reason that avoidance must be for life.

chapter 7

Type IV Hypersensitivity

 CASE 22

Miss Noakes, a 25-year-old lady, consulted a dermatologist after noticing a rash on her right wrist, both ear lobes, and both sides of her neck. She had had acne as a teenager, but had no personal or family history of allergy or atopic dermatitis.

On examination the affected areas consisted of erythema and small blisters. The dermatologist strongly suspected allergic contact dermatitis and questioned Miss Noakes about her use of cosmetics and jewellery. She revealed that she had recently been given a matching bracelet and earring set by her boyfriend and had worn it on several occasions, most recently two days before this consultation.

Patch testing by the application of a battery of commonly implicated agents to the skin of Miss Noakes' back was carried out in the clinic. Examples of agents used included rubber, cosmetics, plant extracts, and metals. Examination of the sites at two and four days after the application showed eczematous reactions to nickel and rubber. Miss Noakes was advised to stop wearing the jewellery and, as an incidental finding, to avoid contact with rubber gloves. She was also prescribed a mild topical corticosteroid for her rash. She had no further episodes of contact dermatitis following this advice.

QUESTIONS

1 What are the characteristics of the 'antigen' in the jewellery?
2 Are there any *in vitro* tests that might be used to make this diagnosis?
3 Can patients be desensitised to contact allergens?
4 Can drugs be contact allergens?

NOTES FOR REVISION

YOUR ANSWERS

1 Characteristics of the 'antigen' in the jewellery

2 *In vitro* tests that might be used to make this diagnosis

3 Can patients be desensitised to contact allergens?

4 Can drugs be contact allergens?

CASE 22

ANSWERS

1 Characteristics of the 'antigen' in the jewellery

The 'antigen' that causes contact hypersensitivity is often a chemical hapten and has to link to body protein before it can become antigenic. Prolonged contact is often necessary for sensitivity to occur: for example, chromate in cement workers after many years of working with it.

2 *In vitro* tests that might be used to make this diagnosis

Lymphocyte transformation, which is a reflection of delayed type hypersensitivity, can be used to demonstrate reactivity to contact allergens including nickel. It is not a practical test and is not used diagnostically.

3 Can patients be desensitised to contact allergens?

It is not practicable to try and desensitise patients to contact antigens although the original experiments of Landsteiner and Chase do suggest that this may be possible.

4 Can drugs be contact allergens?

Drugs can certainly become contact allergens: for example, an antibiotic such as neomycin is a frequent offender. This is seen when a mixture of antibiotic and cortisone cream is used to treat a skin infection. There is an initial healing of the skin, but with repeated application of the cream the lesions get worse. This is due to the induction of Type IV contact allergy to the antibiotic neomycin.

CASE 23

A 15-year-old boy, Kanti, who had recently arrived in the UK from India, consulted his doctor following a three-month history of 'feeling unwell'. Initially his symptoms had been of malaise, reduced appetite, and a weight loss of 3 kg. He had also noticed episodes of fever and sweating at night. More recently he had developed an occasional cough and was breathless on exertion. He had not had any haemoptysis.

On examination Kanti was underweight for his height and age and coughed during the consultation. He had no finger clubbing. His temperature was mildly elevated and his radial pulse was 104 beats/min. Examination of his chest revealed an area of dull percussion note and reduced air entry at the right base with wheezes over the right middle zone. The rest of his cardiovascular examination was normal. The results of investigations are shown in Fig. 7.1.

Fig. 7.1 Results of investigations

Investigation	Result
Chest radiograph	Right hilar enlargement with an area of consolidation in the right middle zone. A small pleural effusion was also present at the right lung base
Red cell count	Normal
White cell count	Normal
ESR (a nonspecific indicator of infection, inflammation, and malignancy)	Raised
Blood cultures	Negative
Sputum microscopy and culture	Positive for *Mycobacterium tuberculosis*
Intradermal injection of purified protein derivative (PPD) of *M. tuberculosis*	Strongly positive Mantoux test

A clear diagnosis of primary tuberculosis infection with pleural effusion was made. Kanti was started on a course of isoniazid and rifampicin (both bactericidal agents) for nine months with ethambutol (a bacteriostatic agent) for the first two months. A subsequent chest radiograph taken at twelve months showed some fibrosis of the right middle lobe, but no evidence of active disease.

QUESTIONS

1 What are the characteristics of an antigen that can lead to granuloma formation?
2 What are the characteristics of a granuloma?
3 Which groups of patients are more prone to infection with *M. tuberculosis*, and why?
4 Can healed tubercular lesions reactivate?

NOTES FOR REVISION

YOUR ANSWERS

1 Characteristics of an antigen that can lead to granuloma formation

2 Characteristics of a granuloma

3 Groups of patients more prone to infection with *M. tuberculosis*, and why?

4 Can healed tubercular lesions reactivate?

CASE 23

pp. 22.1, 22.4–22.6

ANSWERS

1 Characteristics of an antigen that can lead to granuloma formation

To form a granuloma, microorganism or particles that the cell cannot destroy needs to persist within macrophages. This reaction can also be caused by persistent immune complexes: for example, in extrinsic allergic alveolitis. Talc, zirconium, and beryllium can also produce this reaction.

2 Characteristics of a granuloma

The histology of a granuloma is different from that of a tuberculin reaction, which is usually a self-limiting response to an antigen. The epithelioid cell is characteristic of granulomatous hypersensitivity. Multinucleate giant cells are also seen and may be a terminal differentiation step of the monocyte/macrophage line. In non-immunological granulomas, lymphocytes are not seen, thus distinguishing the one from the other.

3 Groups of patients more prone to infection with *M. tuberculosis*, and why?

Those who come into contact with others who do have active tuberculosis and people whose immune system is depressed due to immuno-suppressive drugs or disease, for example AIDS, are more prone to develop TB.

4 Can healed tubercular lesions reactivate?

Mycobacteria can remain alive within a small calcified lymph node. If immunity is altered, for example by long-term corticosteroid therapy, they can be released and lead to re-infection.

CASE 24

At 40 years of age Mr James noticed nodules on his face, arms, and buttocks. At this stage he had no impairment of sensation in any part of his body. Gradually, the skin on his face became thickened and furrowed and the bridge of his nose became flattened. It was decided to start treatment and a few days after the start of the antibiotics he developed a fever, arthralgia, marked malaise, and a leucocytosis. In the next few days he developed red lesions on his legs, which were tender and raised above the surface of the skin. Erythema nodosum leprosum was diagnosed.

QUESTIONS

1 What is the pathogenesis of erythema nodosum leprosum?
2 What is likely to be seen if the lesions are biopsied?
3 What is the mechanism of a borderline leprosy reaction?
4 If severe, how can a borderline leprosy reaction be treated?

NOTES FOR REVISION

OUR ANSWERS

1 Mechanism of erythema nodosum leprosum

2 What is likely to be seen if the lesions are biopsied?

3 Mechanism of a borderline leprosy reaction

4 How can a severe borderline leprosy reaction be treated?

CASE 24

pp. 22.9–22.10

ANSWERS

1 Mechanism of erythema nodosum leprosum

During the course of antibiotic treatment of lepromatous leprosy considerable quantities of leprosy antigen are released into the circulation where they form immune complexes with the already circulating antibody. This results in deposition to give Arthus-type lesions (a Type III hypersensitivity reaction), which lead to erythema nodosum, and also systemic symptoms of fever, lencocytosis and joint pain.

2 What is likely to be seen if the lesions are biopsied?

With immunofluorescence, deposits of immunoglobulin and C3 can be seen in the blood vessel walls, producing a leukocytoclastic vasculitis. This is evidence for the deposition of immune complexes that can fix complement.

3 Mechanism of a borderline leprosy reaction

Where there are *Mycobacterium leprae* organisms in the skin, there is the potential for delayed-type hypersensitivity (DTH) reactions. The increase in DTH can come about naturally or as a result of drug treatment. The skin lesions then become inflamed and swollen and more resemble the tuberculoid form of the disease. This reaction can occur in peripheral nerves and unless treated quickly, nerve destruction occurs because of the ensuing inflammation and fibrosis and small blood vessel obstruction.

4 How can a severe borderline leprosy reaction be treated?

Prompt treatment with corticosteroids.

CASE 25

Mrs Roberts, aged 32, had been feeling unwell for some time, complaining of lethargy, weakness, general malaise, and weight loss. She also had some night sweats and low-grade fever. She then developed some dyspnoea and a cough. A visit to her doctor was precipitated by the appearance of a red and slightly tender rash on the front of her shins which was diagnosed as erythema nodosum. Her joints were also tender and she wondered if she had developed an allergy because of her red eyes. The doctor found that she had a temperature and ordered some investigations. The results are shown in Fig. 7.2.

Fig. 7.2 Results of investigations

Investigation	Result
Chest radiograph	Bilateral hilar lymphadenopathy
Routine blood count	Normal
Serum calcium	Raised

Bronchoscopy and bronchoalveolar lavage were performed. Bronchial lavage showed a lymphocytic alveolitis with predominant CD4$^+$ cells. A diagnosis of sarcoidosis was made.

QUESTIONS

1 What is the aetiology of sarcoidosis?
2 Describe the classification of sarcoidosis?
3 What is the cause of the hypercalcaemia?
4 What is the prognosis of the disease in this patient?

NOTES FOR REVISION

YOUR ANSWERS

1 Aetiology of sarcoidosis

2 Classification of sarcoidosis

3 Cause of the hypercalcaemia

4 Prognosis of the disease in Mrs Roberts

CASE 25

pp. 22.11–22.12

ANSWERS

1 Aetiology of sarcoidosis

Despite the great advances made in understanding the immunopathology of sarcoid, the aetiology is still unknown. The relationship with tuberculosis and other forms of granulomatous conditions is still a matter for discussion, resting on the histopathology of the lesions rather than the aetiological agent.

2 Classification of sarcoidosis

- Type I is characterised by hilar node enlargement, usually bilateral.
- Type II shows hilar gland enlargement with peripheral lung lesions.
- Type III is characterised by parenchymal lung lesions only.

3 Cause of the hypercalcaemia

Hypercalcaemia is present in 10–50% of patients and is a fairly common asymptomatic and transient finding during the active phase of the disease. It appears to result from vitamin D-stimulated intestinal absorption of calcium and is associated with high circulating concentrations of 1,25-dihydroxycholecalciferol, the active form of vitamin D, thought to arise from the conversion of 25-hydroxyvitamin D_3 by pulmonary macrophages.

4 Prognosis of the disease in Mrs Roberts

In general an acute onset indicates a good prognosis. Where the disease has an insidious onset with pulmonary fibrosis, the outlook is less good. Where there is serious hypercalcaemia, treatment with corticosteroids is necessary.

chapter 8

Transplantation and Rejection

■ CASE 26

A 40-year-old lady, Mrs Peacock, was seen in her local hospital after noticing fresh blood in her urine. On questioning she said that she had been feeling unwell for several weeks.

On investigation Mrs Peacock's blood pressure was 150/105 mm Hg and urinalysis demonstrated moderate quantities of protein. Serum urea and creatinine were both moderately raised. Renal biopsies confirmed a diagnosis of rapidly progressive glomerulonephritis.

Despite the use of antihypertensive agents and haemodialysis Mrs Peacock's renal function deteriorated and end-stage renal failure was diagnosed. In order to seek a suitable donor for renal transplantation, she was tissue typed for major histocompatibility antigens (MHC) using anti-HLA antibodies. Her profile was found to be HLA -A10, -A28, -B7, -Bw52, -Cw2, -Cw6, -DR2, -DRw10, with blood group B positive. A suitable cadaveric kidney was found from a donor of HLA type -A9, -A11, -B7, -B17, -Cw2, -Cw8, -DR2, -DR4, and the same blood group.

Transplantation was combined with the triple immunosuppressive regimen of prednisolone, cyclosporin, and azathioprine to aid acceptance of the graft. Serum creatinine and urea levels fell postoperatively and hourly urine output from the graft was satisfactory. Her blood pressure dropped to 140/90 mm Hg.

Five days following the transplant Mrs Peacock developed a fever and was noted to be lethargic. On examination her blood pressure was 155/110 mm Hg and she was tender in the region of the graft. Her urine output had decreased and serum urea and creatinine were raised. An anti-HLA antibody screen was positive. A renal biopsy contained a mononuclear cell infiltrate. Corticosteroid dosages were increased and her renal function recovered transiently, but the graft was eventually rejected.

QUESTIONS
1 Why was the graft rejected so quickly?
2 How has Mrs Peacock developed anti-HLA antibodies?
3 What are the chances of success of a subsequent graft?
4 What is Mrs Peacock's long-term outlook?

NOTES FOR REVISION

YOUR ANSWERS

1 Why the graft was rejected so quickly

2 How Mrs Peacock developed anti-HLA antibodies

3 Chances of success of a subsequent graft

4 Mrs Peacock's long-term outlook

CASE 26

Chapter 23

ANSWERS

1 Why the graft was rejected so quickly

Because anti-HLA antibodies were already circulating with specificity for the graft that the patient had just received, this led to hyperacute rejection, partly due to accelerated platelet agglutination.

2 How Mrs Peacock developed anti-HLA antibodies

The most common mechanism is through pregnancy where the mother becomes sensitised to the father's antigens through transplacental passage of fetal cells.

3 Chances of success of a subsequent graft

There is no reason why a subsequent graft should not be successful if the match is good and particularly avoiding any mismatch, which includes any of the father's HLA antigens.

4 Mrs Peacock's long-term outlook

With a successful graft, the long-term outlook should not be significantly different from other patients receiving a first graft.

chapter 9

Autoimmunity and Autoimmune Disease

▌ CASE 27

Miss Jacob, a 30-year-old Caribbean lady, was seen in a rheumatology clinic with stiff painful joints in her hands, which were worse first thing in the morning. Other symptoms included fatigue, a low-grade fever, a weight loss of 2 kg, and some mild chest pain. Miss Jacob had recently returned to the UK from a holiday in Jamaica and was also noted to be taking the combined oral contraceptive pill. Past medical history of note was a mild autoimmune haemolytic anaemia two years previously.

On examination Miss Jacob had a nonspecific maculopapular rash on her face and chest and patchy alopecia (hair loss) over her scalp. Her mouth was tender and examination revealed an ulcer on the soft palate. She had moderately swollen and tender proximal interphalangeal joints. Her other joints were unaffected, but she had generalised muscle aches. The results of investigations are shown in Fig. 9.1.

Fig. 9.1 Results of investigations

Investigation	Result
Radiograph of hands	Soft-tissue swelling, but no bone erosions
Chest radiograph	A small pleural effusion at the right lung base
Full blood count	A mild normocytic, normochromic anaemia and mild lymphocytopenia
C-reactive protein levels	Normal
Erythrocyte sedimentation rate	Raised
Rheumatoid factor	Negative
Serum IgG levels	Elevated
Antinuclear antibodies (ANA)	Positive by immunofluorescence
Anti-double stranded DNA, anti-RNA, and anti-histone antibodies	Positive by ELISA
Complement (C3 and C4) levels	Low
Skin biopsy from an area unaffected by the rash	Deposition of IgG and complement components at the junction between dermis and epidermis (lupus 'band' test)

A diagnosis of systemic lupus erythematosus (SLE) was made. Miss Jacob was treated with chloroquine, an antimalarial, for the rash on her face and chest.

At a follow-up appointment urinalysis showed protein and red cells. Serum creatinine was mildly elevated as was her blood pressure. A renal biopsy showed membranous lupus nephritis. She was prescribed oral corticosteroids and an antihypertensive agent, which improved her renal function. Her physician also gave advice regarding birth control and pregnancy, and regular check-ups were arranged.

QUESTIONS

1 What is the immunological mechanism leading to the glomerulonephritis?
2 Are immune complexes the main mediator of systemic damage?
3 What is the mechanism for the vasculitis seen in SLE?
4 Are anti-double stranded DNA antibodies pathognomonic of SLE?

YOUR ANSWERS

1 Immunological mechanism leading to the glomerulonephritis

2 Are immune complexes the main mediator of systemic damage?

3 Mechanism for the vasculitis seen in SLE?

4 Are anti-double stranded DNA antibodies pathognomonic of SLE?

CASE 27

pp. 20.9, 21.1, 21.11, 24.2, 24.6, 24.10

ANSWERS

1 Immunological mechanism leading to the glomerulonephritis

It is thought that free DNA filtered in the kidney fixes to the glomerular basement membrane and can then bind anti-DNA antibodies, which then form an immune complex *in situ*. Complement is then fixed, resulting in local damage.

2 Are immune complexes the main mediator of systemic damage?

This is a vexed question. Although DNA–anti-DNA complexes are found in tissues, efforts to find these complexes in the serum have failed. In addition, immunising lupus-prone animals with DNA does not produce clinical lupus. However, introduction of transgenes encoding anti-ds DNA in mice can produce lupus.

3 Mechanism for the vasculitis seen in SLE?

A possible explanation is that the mononuclear-phagocyte system becomes saturated and is therefore unable to clear the soluble complexes, which are thought to be most likely pathogenic. It is also possible that the reduction in the complement receptors on red cells (CR1) might also predispose to poor clearance of complexes.

4 Are anti-double stranded DNA antibodies pathognomonic of SLE?

Over 95% of patients with SLE have ANA as the major autoantibody. Antibodies to extractable nuclear antigens are also seen, but much less frequently. Anti-double stranded DNA antibodies are the most specific to SLE because anti-single stranded antibodies are found in a variety of other situations, such as other autoimmune diseases, a variety of infections, and inflammatory conditions.

CASE 28

A 45-year-old lady, Mrs Smith, visited her doctor after noticing a painless swelling at the front of her neck. On questioning she said that it had taken two to three years to reach its present size. She was otherwise in good health.

On examination Mrs Smith's thyroid was found to be diffusely enlarged and firm, the enlargement including the isthmus of the gland producing a 'butterfly' appearance. She had no signs related to a disturbance of thyroid function.

Measurement of serum T3, T4, and thyroid stimulating hormone (TSH) using specific radioimmunoassays produced results within the normal ranges, demonstrating that Mrs Smith was euthyroid. Serum haemagglutination assays revealed the presence of clinically significant levels of anti-thyroglobulin and anti-thyroid microsomal (anti-thyroid peroxidase) antibodies.

Mrs Smith was referred to a surgeon for consideration of partial thyroid-ectomy. However, before any action could be taken, she returned to her doctor complaining of increasing lethargy and slowness of movement. Her husband noted that her memory recall had deteriorated and that her actions were clumsy. Mrs Smith also noticed that her weight had increased. On discussing her family history she remembered a first degree relative with pernicious anaemia.

On examination Mrs Smith had dry skin, a gruff voice, and a 'puffy' face. Her radial pulse was 55 beats/min. Serum measurements of T3 and T4 were now below the normal ranges. TSH levels were elevated. Re-evaluation of anti-thyroid antibodies showed raised levels compared with the initial results. Mrs Smith was diagnosed as having Hashimoto's thyroiditis and treated with oral thyroxine tablets, which improved her symptoms.

QUESTIONS

1 Is there a genetic predisposition to autoimmune disease?
2 Can autoantibodies to thyroid have different effects on the gland, for example stimulation or inhibition?
3 If diagnosed early enough, should immunosuppressive drugs be given to stop the autoimmune process?
4 Is there an overlap between thyroiditis and other organ-specific autoimmune diseases?

NOTES FOR REVISION

YOUR ANSWERS

1 Is there a genetic predisposition to autoimmune disease?

2 Can autoantibodies to thyroid have different effects on the gland, for example stimulation or inhibition?

3 If diagnosed early enough, should immunosuppressive drugs be given to stop the autoimmune process?

4 Is there an overlap between thyroiditis and other organ-specific autoimmune diseases?

CASE 28

ANSWERS

1 Is there a genetic predisposition to autoimmune disease?

There are definite HLA associations with autoimmune disease, such as DR5 for Hashimoto's disease. Type I diabetes is associated with DR3 and DR4. Thus genes must predispose individuals to develop autoimmunity and also determine which antigens are involved.

2 Can autoantibodies to thyroid have different effects on the gland, for example stimulation or inhibition?

Complement-fixing anti-thyroid peroxidase antibodies are cytotoxic but only if they can gain access to the apical surface of the thyrocyte; others can either block the binding of thyroid stimulating hormone (TSH) or actually stimulate the gland by stimulating another epitope on the TSH receptor itself.

3 If diagnosed early enough, should immunosuppressive drugs be given to stop the autoimmune process?

With a relatively simple condition such as Hashimoto's disease, where oral hormone replacement is so simple, heavy weight immunosuppression is not justified. For diabetics who face a lifetime of injections, this approach in itself may not be optimum, but efforts to control the destruction of the islets or transplant them must be an aim.

4 Is there an overlap between thyroiditis and other organ-specific autoimmune diseases?

There is the classic association of gastritis with thyroiditis. Patients with the one often have autoantibodies to the latter, and vice versa. There is also an association with other organ-specific autoimmune diseases.

CASE 29

When Mrs Booth went for her annual check-up at the age of 42 she was found to be fit, but to have a raised alkaline phosphatase. Other routine investigations at the time showed nothing untoward. Over the next few years her alkaline phosphatase levels increased and she showed a slight, but significant increase in the level of aspartate transaminase and alanine transaminase. Six years later she went to her doctor complaining of itching, and it was then noticed that her bilirubin level was raised. Tests for hepatitis B surface antigen were negative. Mrs Booth later developed a palpable spleen and moderate ascites. Several diagnoses were considered when no evidence of neoplastic disease was found. Eventually, autoantibodies were measured and she was found to have high titres of antimitochondrial antibodies. Liver biopsy was done to confirm the diagnosis of primary biliary cirrhosis.

QUESTIONS

1 What is the mechanism for the damage seen in primary biliary cirrhosis? What is the main site of attack?

2 What other diseases are associated with elevated titres of antimitochondrial antibodies?

3 What is the antigen represented by the antimitochondrial activity?

4 What treatment can be given to patients with primary biliary cirrhosis?

NOTES FOR REVISION

YOUR ANSWERS

1 Mechanism for the damage seen in primary biliary cirrhosis and the main site of attack

2 Other diseases associated with elevated titres of antimitochondrial antibodies

3 The antigen represented by the antimitochondrial activity

4 Treatment for primary biliary cirrhosis

CASE 29

Chapter 24

ANSWERS

1 Mechanism for the damage seen in primary biliary cirrhosis and the main site of attack

The antimitochondrial antibody does not have any direct pathogenetic activity, although anti-M2 sera can cross-react with epitopes on *E. coli*. This may reflect similarities between mitochondrial and bacterial cell membranes. Lymphocytes in the portal tracts are mainly T cells. Both class I and class II molecules are expressed on damaged and normal bile duct epithelium within the same portal tract, which may render the cells vulnerable to attack by cytotoxic T cells.

2 Other diseases associated with elevated titres of antimitochondrial antibodies

A range of liver diseases are associated with raised levels of antimitochondrial antibodies: for example, cryptogenic cirrhosis, chronic active hepatitis, and in a small proportion of cases of biliary obstruction.

3 The antigen represented by the antimitochondrial activity

The antigen, M2, is now known to be a component of the pyruvate dehydrogenase complex and is located on the inner membrane of the mitochondria. The antimitochondrial activity in other diseases is directed against specificities other than the M2 antigen.

4 Treatment for primary biliary cirrhosis

No treatment has been shown to be effective in reversing the bile duct damage. Symptomatic treatment with cholestyramine may be useful.

CASE 30

A 45-year-old lady, Mrs Belcher, was seen by her doctor with symptoms of increasing pain and stiffness in her wrists and fingers. Several years previously she had experienced similar symptoms, but they had receded during her last pregnancy. She stated that since the birth of the child she had found it progressively more awkward to knit (her favourite pastime). The stiffness was worse in the morning, although her hands felt clumsy throughout the day. Recently she had also noticed a tingling sensation in the thumb and first two fingers of both hands, which was worse at night.

On examination Mrs Belcher had tender swellings at her wrist, proximal inter-phalangeal, and metacarpophalangeal joints, the latter being most marked. Ulnar deviation of the fingers was also present and she was unable to clench either hand to make a fist. There was no evidence of any muscle wasting and no further joints were involved. Respiratory, cardiovascular, and neurological examinations were all normal. The results of investigations are shown in Fig. 9.2.

Fig. 9.2 Results of investigations

Investigation	Result
Haemoglobin	Normal
White cell count	Normal
Levels of C-reactive protein (CRP)	Elevated
Latex agglutination assay to detect IgM rheumatoid factor (RF)	Negative
Antinuclear antibodies	Not detected
Serum complement (C3 and C4) levels	Normal

A diagnosis of early rheumatoid arthritis was made and Mrs Belcher was prescribed aspirin. This initially provided some relief of her symptoms, but also caused gastric irritation. She returned to her doctor three months later with worsening symptoms in her hands and involvement of both her knees.

On examination her metacarpophalangeal joints were swollen and very tender. Effusions were present in both her knees. Indomethacin was prescribed to control the effusions and the aspirin was discontinued.

Nine months after first visiting her doctor Mrs Belcher developed bilateral subcutaneous nodules on the extensor surfaces of her forearms. The tingling sensation in her hands that she had described at her first visit had progressed to shooting pains alternating with numbness. The power in her abductus pollicis brevis muscle was reduced and wasting was evident. Palmar erythema was noted bilaterally. The nodules on her arms were 1 cm in diameter, firm, mobile, and non-tender. Serum analysis was now positive for RF and negative for antinuclear antibodies. She had a moderate microcytic anaemia, but a normal white cell count. CRP levels were raised and complement was normal. Radiographic examination of her wrists and hands showed erosions at the distal radii and the metacarpophalangeal joints. Mrs Belcher's drug treatment was changed to ibuprofen and she was referred for physiotherapy.

QUESTIONS

1 What is the significance of the subcutaneous nodules?
2 What is Mrs Belcher's long-term prognosis?
3 What other drugs are available for treatment of her rheumatoid arthritis?
4 Is lung involvement likely?

YOUR ANSWERS

1 Significance of the subcutaneous nodules

2 Mrs Belcher's long-term prognosis

3 Other drugs available for treating Mrs Belcher's rheumatoid arthritis

4 Is lung involvement likely?

CASE 30

pp. 9.12, 21.9–21–10, 24.2

ANSWERS

1 Significance of the subcutaneous nodules

Subcutaneous nodules are found in patients who are seropositive and are usually associated with high levels of RF and a more severe course of the disease. They occur in 20–30% of patients.

2 Mrs Belcher's long-term prognosis

Mrs Belcher's disease is progressing quite rapidly and in view of the presence of nodules and high levels of RF the prognosis is not that good.

3 Other drugs available for treating Mrs Belcher's rheumatoid arthritis

A number of different anti-inflammatory compounds are available for treatment and can be given with other drugs such as gold, D-penicillamine, antimalarials, immunosuppressives and corticosteroids.

4 Is lung involvement likely?

Lung involvement in RA is not common and was thought to be mainly of the restrictive type. It is now thought that some of the lung involvement may be obstructive in character.

CASE 31

Miss Heller, a 25-year-old North German lady, was admitted to hospital with a history of fatigue, myalgia, diffuse abdominal pain, anorexia, and amenorrhoea. She had no history of intravenous drug abuse and no family history of malignancy or liver disease. Past medical history of note was hypothyroidism diagnosed five years earlier for which she was receiving thyroxine supplements. She was not on any other medication.

On examination Miss Heller had palmar erythema, numerous spider naevi, hepatosplenomegaly, and was clearly jaundiced. No Kayser–Fleisher rings were seen. The results of investigations are shown in Fig. 9.3.

Fig. 9.3 Results of investigations

Investigation	Result
Serum aspartate aminotransferase	Raised
Serum alanine aminotransferase	Raised
Serum bilirubin	Mild conjugated hyperbilirubinaemia
Alkaline phosphatase	Normal
Serum albumin	Normal
Prothrombin time	Prolonged
Anti-HBc IgM	Negative
White cell count	Normal
Haemoglobin	10.0 g/dl (low)
IgG	Elevated
IgA and IgM	Normal
Antinuclear antibodies, anti-smooth muscle antibodies, and anti-dsDNA antibodies	Positive
Liver biopsy	Piecemeal necrosis and evidence of cirrhosis. T cells and plasma cells identified by immunohistochemistry

A diagnosis of autoimmune chronic active hepatitis (CAH) was made and Miss Heller was started on corticosteroid and vitamin K therapy. Within a fortnight her liver function test results had returned to normal and her symptoms had improved. She was discharged on a maintenance dosage of corticosteroids and was reviewed regularly.

QUESTIONS
1 What are the possible causes for this condition?
2 What are the immunological mechanisms of damage?
3 What treatment should be given?
4 What are the main differences between the two major types of CAH?

YOUR ANSWERS

1 Possible causes

2 Immunological mechanisms

3 Treatment

4 Main differences between the two major types of CAH

NOTES FOR REVISION

CASE 31

p. 24.2

ANSWERS

1 Possible causes

In cases where no obvious cause is found, the autoimmune form is suspected. Of the definable conditions, CAH can be associated with HBsAg, drugs, alpha-1 antitrypsin deficiency, and Wilson's disease.

2 Immunological mechanisms

The immunopathology is complex, but antibody, K cell cytotoxicity, and T cell responses to liver-specific membrane lipoprotein (LSP) have all been described. T cell sensitisation to a component of the LSP, a receptor for a sialoglycoprotein is characteristic of all patients with CAH.

3 Treatment

The treatment of the autoimmune form is to suppress whichever mechanism is leading to the autoimmune cell damage. Corticosteroids reduce the inflammatory response and produce clinical remission. Although there is less cellular infiltrate with this treatment, cirrhosis is not halted. Immunosuppressive drugs will reduce the need for corticosteroids. If CAH is associated with a viral infection, interferon-alpha has been shown to be helpful.

4 Main differences between the two major types of CAH

See Fig. 9.4 (adapted from Chapel and Haeney, *Essentials of Clinical Immunology,* 3rd edn, Blackwells, 12.11).

Fig. 9.4 Major differences between the two main types of CAH

Feature	Autoimmune CAH	Hepatitis B and C associated CAH
Proportion of all cases of CAH in the UK	50–80%	20–50%
Sex	85% female	90% male
Age at onset	10–30 years 40–60 years	Elderly
Associated autoimmune disease	Common	Rare
Smooth muscle antibodies	Positive in 70%	Low titre or absent
Antinuclear antibodies	Positive in 80%	Negative
Anti-DNA antibodies	May be positive	Negative
Antimitochondrial antibodies	Positive in 25%	Negative
Antibodies to liver and kidney microsomes	May be positive (especially in children)	Negative
Serum immunoglobulins	IgG ↑↑	Normal or IgG ↑
HLA type	HLA-B8,-DR3	?
Response to corticosteroids	Good	?
Risk of hepatoma	Low	High

CASE 32

When Lucy went to her doctor complaining of feeling tired she was told that it was just the studying for University entrance that was the cause. Her doctor did not bother to examine her. She went back to him in the school holidays complaining of increased tiredness, muscle weakness, some abdominal problems, and sweats. He did examine her on this occasion and found her blood pressure to be low at 95/60 mm Hg and noted that she did seem to have a good sun tan. In her family her mother had thyroid disease and an aunt was recently diagnosed as an insulin-dependent diabetic. Further examination showed pigmentation of Lucy's nail beds, areolae, gum margins, and buccal mucosa.

A plain abdominal radiograph was normal. Biochemical tests showed deficient production of both glucocorticoids and mineralocorticoids. Autoantibodies were positive to adrenal cortex cytoplasm of the zona granulosa and fasciculata. A diagnosis of Addison's disease was made.

QUESTIONS

1 What is the evidence for immune involvement in autoimmune Addison's disease?
2 What other endocrine diseases are associated with this form of Addison's disease?
3 What used to be the major cause of Addison's disease?
4 What treatment should be given?

YOUR ANSWERS

1 Evidence for immune involvement in autoimmune Addison's disease

2 Other endocrine diseases associated with this form of Addison's disease

3 Major cause of Addison's disease in the past

4 Treatment

NOTES FOR REVISION

CASE 32

p. 24.2

ANSWERS

1 Evidence for immune involvement in autoimmune Addison's disease

There is an association with other autoimmune diseases. There is a high incidence of other organ-specific autoantibodies and also antibodies to the steroid cells of the adrenal cortex. *In vitro* cell-mediated immunity shows reaction of lymphocytes to adrenal cortical tissue. Experimentally, immunisation with adrenal tissue in complete Freund's adjuvant and passive transfer of cells from immunised animals can lead to adrenal failure.

2 Other endocrine diseases associated with this form of Addison's disease

Almost 50% of patients have another autoimmune disease, such as thyroiditis, diabetes mellitus, ovarian failure, or pernicious anaemia.

3 Major cause of Addison's disease in the past

Tuberculous infection of the adrenal gland used to be the main cause of hormonal failure in Addison's disease. This is now rare.

4 Treatment

Replacement therapy as indicated by the biochemical tests. In spite of a high level of autoantibodies and some destruction of the adrenal gland, there is sometimes a compensatory increase in ACTH which may maintain gland function despite increasing cell damage.

CASE 33

When David was 14 years old he started to complain of pains in his joints and in his back. The doctor could find no significant abnormality when he examined him and a full blood count was normal. The pains got worse and it became more difficult for David to get out of bed in the morning because of the stiffness. Blood tests again showed no abnormality other than a raised ESR of 32 mm/hr.

David was then seen by a rheumatologist. On examination he found that David's spine was slightly bowed, his hips lacked mobility, his knees and heels were painful, and he had a mild iritis. The results of investigations are shown in Fig. 9.5.

Fig. 9.5 Results of investigations

Investigation	Result
Rheumatoid factor assays	Negative
Radiographs	Classic changes associated with ankylosing spondylitis, i.e. fused sacro-iliac joints and 'bamboo spine'
Tissue typing	HLA B27

Exercise and anti-inflammatory drugs relieved many, but not all, of the symptoms. David was then put on a low carbohydrate diet and within a few weeks he felt very much better and his ESR had returned to normal levels. Total IgA was increased and antibodies to *Klebsiella pneumoniae* were present in high titre. These returned to more normal levels after some months on the diet.

QUESTIONS

1 What percentage of patients with ankylosing spondylitis (AS) are HLA B27 positive?
2 What is the significance of antibodies to *Klebsiella pneumoniae*?
3 Can other organisms be associated with seronegative spondylarthropathies?
4 Could this disease be caused by molecular mimicry? If so, what experiments might you do to investigate this possibility?

NOTES FOR REVISION

YOUR ANSWERS

1 Percentage of patients with ankylosing spondylitis who are HLA B27 positive

2 Significance of antibodies to *Klebsiella pneumoniae*

3 Can other organisms be associated with seronegative spondylarthropathies?

4 Could this disease be caused by molecular mimicry? If so, what experiments might you do to investigate this possibility?

CASE 33

pp.24.8–24.11

ANSWERS

1 Percentage of patients with ankylosing spondylitis who are HLA B27 positive

Ankylosing spondylitis is the purest form of spondylarthritis, with 95% of the patients being HLA B27 positive, in contrast to a low frequency (around 8%) of HLA B27 in the Caucasian population. This phenotype is useful for the diagnosis, as AS is unlikely to be present in a patient who does not have B27.

2 Significance of antibodies to *Klebsiella pneumoniae*

Two-thirds of patients with AS have subclinical inflammatory gut lesions, supporting the idea that the disease is due to a persisting organism in the gut. Patients have a high level of IgA and high levels of antibodies to *Klebsiella pneumoniae*. When patients start a specific elimination diet with low carbohydrate, the levels of total IgA and antibody to *Klebsiella* fall and this is associated with a clinical improvement. The low-carbohydrate diet leads to a reduction in the levels of *Klebsiella* in the gut.

3 Can other organisms be associated with seronegative spondyloarthropathies?

As two-thirds of the patients have subclinical inflammatory gut lesions, it is clear clinically that other arthritides follow infection in patients who are B27 positive. Organisms commonly associated with reactive arthritis include *Salmonellae, Shigella,* and *Yersinia,* or *Chlamydia* in non-specific urethritis. The arthritis is similar to AS, but tends to be less persistent.

4 Could this disease be caused by molecular mimicry? If so, what experiments might you do to investigate this possibility?

The similarity of the B27 epitope and surface antigens on *Klebsiella pneumoniae* can be shown by absorption experiments or by cross labelling. Purified antibody to *Klebsiella* preferentially stains cells that are HLA B27 positive. The reverse is also the case. This is an example of molecular mimicry and may be playing a role in the pathogenesis of the disease.

Index

A

Acetylcholine receptor antibodies 43–44
Acquired immunodeficiency syndrome (AIDS) 23–24
Addison's disease 71–72
Adrenaline 29, 31
Adult respiratory distress syndrome 11–12
AIDS 23–24
Allergy
    allergic asthma 33–34
    contact dermatitis 51–52
    extrinsic allergic alveolitis 45–46
    genetics 34
    IgA deficiency 18
    penicillin 29–30
Alveolitis
    extrinsic allergic 45–46
    lymphocytic 57
Anaemia
    autoimmune haemolytic 41–42
    multiple myeloma 16
Anaphylactic shock
    bee venom 31–32
    penicillin 29–30
Anaphylatoxins 32
Angioedema, hereditary 27–28
Ankylosing spondylitis 73–74
Anti-D antibodies 39–40
Anti-DNA antibodies 62
Anti-glomerular basement membrane antibodies 37
Anti-HLA antibodies 60
Anti-thyroid antibodies 63
Antibody-coated red blood cells 10
Antigliadin antibodies 50
Antimalarial drugs 68
Antimitochondrial antibodies 66
Arthritis
    hypogammaglobulinaemia 20
    reactive 74
    rheumatoid 67–68
Aspergillus 25
Aspirin 67
Asthma, allergic (extrinsic) 33–34
Autoimmune haemolytic anaemia 41–42
Azathioprine 59

B

B cells 24
Basophils 34
Bee stings 31–32
Bence–Jones protein 16
Benzylpenicillin allergy 29–30
Beta-2 receptor agonists 34

Bird Fancier's lung 46
Blood transfusion 18, 39–40

C

C1 inhibitor 28
C3 deposits 14
Candidiasis, oral 22, 23
Cellulitis 19
Chlamydia spp. 74
Chlorambucil 42
Chloroquine 61
Chlorpheniramine 29, 31
Cholestyramine 66
Choline esterase inhibitors 43–44
Chronic granulomatous disease 25–26
Cirrhosis, primary biliary 65–66
Co-trimoxazole (sulphamethoxazole and
    trimethoprim) 20, 23, 25, 47–48
Coeliac disease (gluten enteropathy) 49–50
Cold haemagglutinin disease 41–42
Contact hypersensitivity 51–52
Corticosteroids 33–34, 37, 45, 56, 58, 61, 68, 69–70
Cyclophosphamide 37
Cyclosporin 36, 59

D

Danazol 28
Dapsone 50
Dermatitis, contact 51–52
Dermatitis herpetiformis 49–50
Desensitisation therapy 30, 31–32, 52
Diabetes mellitus 35–36
DiGeorge syndrome 21–22
Direct antiglobulin test 42
Dobutamine 11
Dopamine 11

E

Encephalitis 20
Endotoxins 12
Epsilon amino caproic acid 28
Epstein–Barr virus 14, 42
Erythema nodosum 57
Erythema nodosum leprosum 55–56
Escherichia coli 11, 66
Ethambutol 53
Extrinsic allergic alveolitis 45–46

F

Farmer's lung 45–46
Fetal thymus transplant 21

Revision notes

Revision notes

Revision notes